CHAIR YOGA
FOR SENIORS
OVER 60

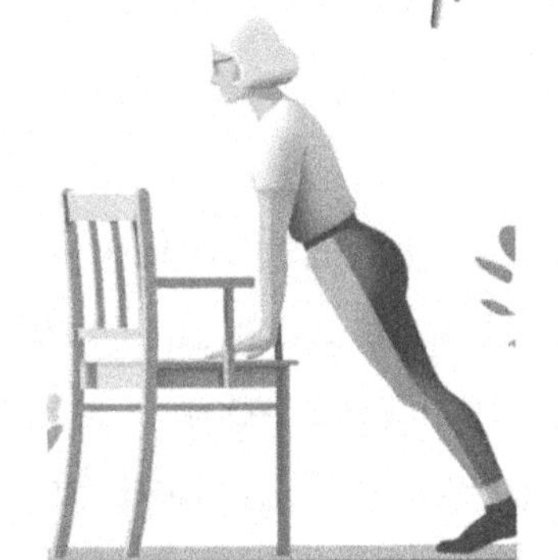

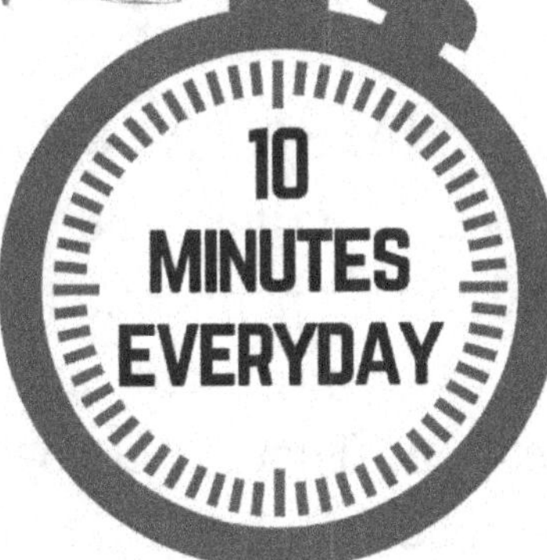

FULLY ILLUSTRATED LOW IMPACT EXERCISES TO IMPROVE MOBILITY, BALANCE AND POSTURE. YOUR WORKOUT GUIDE TO RECLAIM YOUR INDEPENDENCE WITH 28-DAY CHALLENGE

JEREMY LIAM

Hey there! Wow, I'm genuinely over the moon that you've decided to bring this book into your life. Isn't it exciting to think about all the wonderful changes we're about to embark on together?

Thank you so much for trusting me to guide you through the world of chair yoga. Over the years, I've had the joy of helping countless individuals just like you overcome challenges with flexibility, balance, and yes, even weight loss—all through the gentle power of chair yoga. Now, are you ready to improve your flexibility, boost your balance, enhance your posture, and shed those extra pounds? Well, you've chosen the right companion! Chair yoga has worked wonders for many seniors, bringing joy and vitality back into their routines, and now, it's your turn.

How does starting your day feeling stretched out and stress-free sound? Or what about regaining strength in places you haven't felt in years? Together, we'll laugh, stretch, and maybe challenge ourselves a bit. But don't worry—I'll be with you every step (and stretch!) of the way.

So, what do you say, ready to unroll that yoga mat and place your chair? Let's make every movement count and have a ton of fun while we're at it. You won't regret picking up this book—I promise you that!

With all my gratitude and excitement I genuinely hope to fulfill your vacuum in this book

"Physical fitness is the first requisite of happiness."

[Joseph Pilates]

THIS CHAIR YOGA BOOK BELONGS TO

SPECIAL 3-IN-1 GOODIES EXCLUSIVELY IN THE PAPERBACK VERSION!

Hey there! Did you know that enhancing your health goes beyond just practicing yoga poses? That's right! In the paperback version of this book I've included a fantastic 3-in-1 bonus to make your experience even more rewarding. And who doesn't love a good bonus?

1. 28-DAY CHALLENGE: Are you up for a challenge? I designed this 28-Day Challenge to jump-start your chair yoga practice and establish wellness as a daily habit. Each day brings a new opportunity for growth and fun. Are you ready to commit to 28 days of enhancing your well-being?

2. MEAL PLAN: Looking for healthy, easy-to-prepare meals that complement your yoga practice? I've got you covered! This meal plan is packed with delicious recipes that support weight loss and boost your energy. Who said healthy eating has to be boring?

3. PROGRESS TRACKER JOURNAL: Curious about how your chair yoga poses are improving your flexibility, balance, and overall wellness? With the Progress Tracker Journal, you can keep tabs on each pose, monitor your improvements, and really see how far you've come. Are you ready to track your progress and celebrate your achievements?

This exclusive bonus is only available in the paperback version, making it the perfect choice for those who love having a physical book to hold, read, and write in. Plus, it's ideal for jotting down notes and tracking your journey!

So, are you ready to take your health and wellness to the next level with these exciting bonuses? Let's make it fun, let's make it impactful, and let's do it together!

Grab your paperback copy today and let's kick off this exciting adventure. I can't wait to see how much you'll achieve!

DO I EVEN NEED TO DO CHAIR YOGA AS A SENIOR?

Before going further, let's chat about why chair yoga is the ideal fit for your lifestyle, especially as we embrace our golden years. Have you tried asking if you really need chair yoga to improve your health as a senior or is it just one of the trends?
Well, chair yoga is a wonderful adaptation of traditional yoga that makes it accessible, safe, and incredibly beneficial for seniors.

Firstly, chair yoga is super low impact, making it perfect for maintaining joint health and reducing the risk of injury. It's all about achieving physical health without the strain pretty great, right? Now, think about this: have you ever hesitated to try yoga because it seemed too demanding? Well, chair yoga offers all the benefits without any of the stress.a

But don't let the word "gentle" fool you. Chair yoga can help you lose weight and manage your health effectively. How about improving your flexibility, balance, and posture? This form of yoga is tailored to enhance these aspects with each session, helping you move better and feel stronger every day.

Imagine gaining the flexibility to bend down and tie your shoes without a struggle, or improving your balance to walk confidently on uneven paths. Exciting, isn't it? Chair yoga makes all this possible in a fun and supportive way, encouraging you every step of the way.

It's not just about the physical benefits. Practicing yoga from a chair also brings mental clarity and emotional calmness. Ever felt overwhelmed and needed a quick stress relief? A few minutes of chair yoga can be incredibly soothing.

Isn't it time you gave yourself the gift of better health and increased mobility? I will leave to you go think about it.

WHY SHOULD I CHOOSE THIS BOOK?

If you're pondering why this chair yoga book should be your go-to guide, let me share some highlights that make it stand out, especially tailored for someone as splendid as you.

This book is crafted with you in mind focusing on gentle exercises that fit perfectly into the lifestyle of seniors or anyone with limited mobility. Each exercise is designed to ensure you can perform it comfortably and safely, helping you maintain your health without any strain. Isn't it wonderful to find a fitness routine that respects your body's needs?

Now, let's talk about ease of use. Ever felt frustrated with exercise instructions that seem more like a puzzle? Well, no more confusion! This book lays out each pose with clear, easy-to-follow instructions and illustrations that make starting your practice straightforward. Imagine having a friendly guide right beside you, showing you exactly what to do, that's what you can expect.

But that's not all. How does a special 3-in-1 bonus sound? Included exclusively in the paperback version, you'll find a 28-Day Challenge to kick-start your journey, a Meal Plan to support your physical activities with nourishing recipes, and a Progress Tracker Journal to observe your advancements. Each bonus is designed to enhance your experience and maximize your results. Exciting, isn't it, to think about tracking your progress and seeing real improvements?

Why not let this book be your companion on a path to better health and increased vitality? Embrace a life where every movement is a step toward feeling your best, and make fitness a joyful part of your day with a splash of fun and loads of encouragement!

HOW TO USE THIS BOOK

Ready for your new chair yoga adventure ? Whether you're a seasoned yogi or just starting out, this book is designed to make your experience as enriching and enjoyable as possible. Let's walk through how to get the most out of this guide.

Getting Started
First things first, do you have a comfortable chair? Make sure it's sturdy and doesn't have wheels. Safety first! Now, find a quiet spot where you can stretch out a bit your living room, a bedroom, or any space where you feel relaxed.

Navigating the Book
Each chapter of this book is laid out in a way that gradually builds your knowledge and skills. Start at the beginning to understand the basics of chair yoga and its benefits. Have you ever wondered why each pose is beneficial? You'll find the answers here, along with easy-to-follow instructions and illustrations for each exercise.

Daily Practice
How much time can you dedicate to practice? Even a few minutes can make a big difference! Try to establish a routine that fits into your daily schedule. Morning, noon, or night what works best for you?

Using the Bonuses
Don't forget about the special 3-in-1 bonus in the paperback version. Have you checked out the 28-Day Challenge, or started using the Progress Journal Tracker to monitor your improvements? These tools are great for keeping you motivated and engaged.

Listen to Your Body
It's important to listen to your body and adjust the exercises according to your comfort level. Never push into pain, and take breaks whenever you need to. How are you feeling during the exercises? Remember, each stretch should feel good.

Stay Consistent

Consistency is key to seeing results. Try to use this book regularly, even if it's just for a short session each day. Have you noticed any improvements in how you feel after a few sessions?

Share Your Experience

Once you've spent some time with the book, I'd love to hear about your experiences! What's been your favorite pose so far? Sharing your story could inspire others to start their chair yoga journey, too.

Thank you for choosing this book to guide you through your chair yoga practice. Ready to start feeling your best? Let's do this together!

TABLE OF CONTENTS

INTRODUCTION

"Your body is your most precious asset; nurture it with movement, fuel it with love, and watch as it transforms into a vessel of power and grace."

Jeremy Liam

As we progress through the later years of life, finding effective ways to stay active and healthy becomes crucial. That's where chair yoga comes in it's a fantastic option for staying fit and flexible without the strain of traditional workouts.

I've been both practicing and teaching chair yoga for many years, and I've seen the amazing impact it can have. It's not just about keeping fit; it's about enhancing your life with better mobility, less discomfort, and even managing your weight. Imagine being able to improve your physical health and mental well-being in a way that's adapted just for you.

Chair yoga is designed with accessibility in mind. No matter your current level of fitness or mobility, there's a way to adapt each pose to meet your needs. Ever wondered if you could still get the benefits of yoga if you can't manage those complicated floor poses? Chair yoga is the answer, providing support with a chair so you can perform each movement safely and effectively.

Why is chair yoga so beneficial, especially as you get older? It focuses on flexibility, strength, balance, and weight management all things that become more important as we age. The mental boost is a big plus, too. Many of my students report feeling less stressed and more at peace after our sessions. Could this be what you need to bring a new sense of calm and control into your life?

Throughout this book, we'll dive into all the basics you need to get started: from picking the right chair to mastering breathing techniques that enhance your practice. We're not just doing exercises; we're creating a routine that enriches your life.

So, are you ready to join me on this path? You see, let me tell you the story of two of my students I have the opportunity to guide through this successful chair routine. With age our bodies undergo significant changes that can impact how injuries affect us and the dangers of being overweight. Tissues repair more slowly, muscle mass decreases, and the body's metabolic rate declines. These factors mean that recovery from injury can be extended and more complex, and excess weight adds additional stress on joints and organs, elevating the risk of conditions such as arthritis, diabetes, and heart disease. One of my student, a 56-year-old man who led a mostly inactive lifestyle and was significantly overweight, is a prime example of these challenges. He struggled with limited mobility, poor balance and coordination, weak core strength, and limited flexibility. The intensity of traditional exercises was daunting and discouraging, further complicating his situation.

When I met him, I introduced him to chair yoga, a gentle yet effective form of exercise tailored to meet the needs of older adults and those with physical limitations. To ensure a structured approach, we implemented a 28-day challenge workout planner, which included daily activities that gradually increased in intensity at a manageable pace. Alongside this, a specific meal plan aimed at improving his nutritional intake and a progress tracker journal to monitor his daily achievements and reflections played a crucial role in his journey toward better health.

The transformation was profound. Chair yoga not only helped improve his balance and core strength, reducing his risk of falls and common injuries, but it also aided in weight loss and boosted his mental well-being. Motivated by his progress, his 62-year-old friend, who faced similar health challenges, joined him. Together, they took on the 28-day challenge, supporting each other and meticulously documenting their progress in their journals.

Their story is a perfect illustration of the philosophy of chair yoga as we've introduced in the beginning of this book. The combination of the exercise regimen, meal plan, and progress journal tracker highlighted the benefits of a structured health approach in later life, demonstrating that with the right support and adaptations, improving one's quality of life is always possible. This method not only addresses the physical aspects of health but also overcomes the mental barriers that often prevent seniors from adopting a more active lifestyle.

Through chair yoga, both individuals discovered a path to a healthier, more active lifestyle despite the challenges posed by aging and excess weight. Their stories is an evidence to human adaptability and resilience and underscores the importance of fitness programs that respect the body's limits while gently enhancing its capabilities.

CHAPTER 1

EMBRACING CHAIR YOGA AT 60 AND BEYOND

"In 10 sessions you'll feel the difference, in 20 sessions you'll see the difference, and in 30 sessions you'll have a whole new body."
[Joseph Pilates]

Isn't it incredible how reaching 60 can open up new avenues rather than closing them? Chair yoga is one of those fantastic opportunities that allows us to stay active and maintain our health without overtaxing our bodies. For many who hit the senior years, traditional exercise can become a challenge, often due to joint pain or balance issues. That's where chair yoga comes in as a savior—a gentler form of yoga that keeps us moving and flexible.

When you think about exercise, you might not immediately picture doing yoga in a chair, but it's surprisingly effective! Chair yoga involves performing yoga poses while seated or using a chair for support, making it accessible for those who have mobility concerns or who might not feel stable enough for standing poses. The best part? It significantly enhances flexibility, strengthens muscles, and improves posture, helping with everyday activities and overall health.

Beyond the physical, chair yoga works wonders for the mind. Have you ever felt stressed and found that a simple walk or a moment of quiet breathing made all the difference? Well, chair yoga offers this peace and more, reducing anxiety, lifting mood, and overall enhancing well-being. It's not just about the physical moves but also about calming the mind and staying sharp and focused.

Now, think about the community aspect. Starting chair yoga at 60 or older introduces you to a group of peers who are all on a similar path. It's a wonderful way to meet new friends and stay connected, which can be a huge boost to your spirits. Plus, the confidence you gain from improving your balance and coordination is invaluable, not just for preventing falls, which are a common concern at this age, but also for encouraging a more active, independent lifestyle.

So, stepping into chair yoga as you enter your 60s and beyond is really about embracing a healthier, more vibrant lifestyle. It's a safe, enjoyable, and deeply beneficial way to look after both your body and mind. Whether you're aiming to manage stress, keep your independence, or just stay active, chair yoga fits the bill perfectly. How about giving it a try and seeing how much more enjoyable your days can become?

Moreover, let's consider the importance of a routine. As you weave chair yoga into your daily schedule, it will become a treasured part of your routine, something you look forward to not just for the physical exercise but for the peace and joy it brings.

By the end of this book, you'll have a comprehensive grasp of how chair yoga can play a crucial role in your life. You won't just be reading about the changes; you'll be experiencing them. Ready to start feeling better in every way? Let's begin this wonderful practice and discover where it can lead us together!

THE FUNDAMENTALS OF YOGA AND ITS ADAPTATION TO THE CHAIR

Yoga has been celebrated for centuries for its profound impact on health and well-being, blending physical postures, breathing techniques, and meditation. But how does this ancient practice translate into something as modern and accessible as chair yoga, especially designed for seniors? It's all about adapting these time-honored techniques to fit the needs of those who may find traditional yoga poses too challenging.

Let's start with the basics: the core principles of yoga focus on enhancing flexibility, building strength, and promoting mental clarity through controlled movements and breathwork. In chair yoga, these principles are fully intact, but the methods are modified. Instead of standing poses, which may pose a risk of strain or falls for some seniors, chair yoga introduces modified poses that can be done while seated or using a chair for support.

These adaptations make yoga accessible to a broader range of individuals, especially those with limited mobility, balance issues, or chronic pain. For example, a standard yoga pose like the Warrior can be transformed into a seated version that still stretches the hips and strengthens the thighs, but without the need for standing balance.

Breathing remains a crucial element of yoga, even in its chair-adapted form. We teach techniques that focus on expanding the lungs and improving circulation, which are vital for maintaining heart health and reducing anxiety. These techniques are simple yet effective and can be practiced anywhere, anytime.

Moreover, the adaptation of yoga to the chair doesn't just cater to physical limitations. It also opens up the mental and emotional benefits of yoga to those who might otherwise feel excluded from the practice. Meditation and mindfulness are incorporated into chair yoga sessions, helping seniors find mental clarity and emotional peace, enhancing overall quality of life.

In the chapters that follow, we will explore each of these elements in detail. We'll break down specific poses and sequences, discuss the best practices for breath control and meditation, and show how these can be integrated into everyday life. This journey will not only teach you about the fundamentals of chair yoga but also demonstrate how to customize this practice to fit your personal health needs and lifestyle.

ROOTS OF YOGA: UNDERSTANDING ITS CORE PHILOSOPHY

Yoga is more than just a series of poses it's a rich tradition with deep philosophical roots that date back thousands of years in ancient India. Understanding the core philosophy of yoga can enrich your practice and offer deeper insights into the ways it can improve your life, especially as you adapt these teachings to the context of chair yoga.

At its heart, yoga is about union—the term "yoga" itself derives from the Sanskrit word for "yoke," signifying the joining of body, mind, and spirit. This holistic approach is central to yoga philosophy, emphasizing balance and harmony within oneself and with the surrounding world. The foundational text of yoga, the Yoga Sutras, authored by the sage Patanjali, outlines the Eight Limbs of Yoga. These limbs provide a framework for living a meaningful and purposeful life. They include ethical standards, self-discipline, posture practice, breath control, sensory withdrawal, concentration, meditation, and eventual enlightenment. While some aspects focus on the physical, others dive deep into mental and spiritual growth.

In chair yoga, we adapt these principles to make them accessible. For instance, while the physical postures (asanas) are modified to be performed with a chair, the essence of each pose the focus and the breath work remains consistent with traditional practices. This adaptation ensures that even those with physical limitations can enjoy the benefits of yoga, respecting their bodies' needs while still challenging themselves in safe ways.

Breath control (pranayama), another key element, is profoundly beneficial. It helps regulate the body's energy through controlled breathing techniques, leading to better health and a calmer mind. Even seated, these practices can be incredibly powerful, aiding in stress reduction and mental clarity, which are crucial for maintaining quality of life as we age.

Understanding and integrating the core philosophy of yoga into chair yoga practices not only enhances the physical benefits but also enriches the mental and emotional experience. It turns each session into an opportunity for personal reflection and growth, enabling a deeper connection to the self and the broader universe.

Today, chair yoga have become a bridge that connects us to a timeless tradition, empowering us to lead fuller, more balanced lives well into our senior years. Whether you're looking to strengthen your body, soothe your mind, or connect more deeply with your spirit, the comprehensive approach of yoga offers valuable tools to assist you on this path.

THE CHAIR YOGA ADVANTAGE: SAFETY AND ADAPTABILITY

Chair yoga presents a unique blend of safety and adaptability, making it an ideal choice for those who may find traditional yoga practices out of reach. This form of yoga, designed with a chair either as a tool or support, allows individuals to experience the benefits of yoga without the risk associated with more physically demanding postures.

One of the most significant advantages of chair yoga is safety. As we age or face physical limitations, the risk of falls or injuries can increase significantly. Chair yoga minimizes these risks by providing a stable support system—the chair. Whether it's used for sitting or standing poses, the chair offers balance and stability, allowing practitioners to focus on their movements and alignment without the fear of falling. This makes it possible for individuals with balance issues, chronic pain, or those recovering from surgery to safely participate in yoga, improving their strength and flexibility at their own pace.

Adaptability is another cornerstone of chair yoga. Traditional yoga poses are incredibly versatile, and when modified for chair yoga, they become accessible to people of all fitness levels and mobility ranges. For instance, a forward bend can be adapted by remaining seated and extending the torso over the legs, still achieving the stretch along the spine and hamstrings but without the strain of a full standing pose. This adaptability not only caters to physical needs but also respects the personal comfort and safety of each practitioner.

Chair yoga is not just physically adaptable; it's also versatile in terms of where it can be practiced. It's suitable for a variety of settings, from a yoga studio to a home or even an office. Practitioners can grab a few moments of yoga during a break at work or engage in a full session at home, integrating wellness into their daily routine in a convenient way.

The practice also adapts to serve different therapeutic goals. Whether the aim is to reduce stress, manage pain, or improve heart health, chair yoga offers a range of breathing exercises, meditative practices, and physical postures that can be tailored to achieve these health objectives. This aspect of chair yoga is particularly beneficial, as it aligns with the holistic approach of yoga, addressing not just physical but also mental and emotional well-being.

Chair yoga advantage lies in its ability to maintain the integrity and goals of traditional yoga while adapting to the specific needs and conditions of a broader audience. It underscores the philosophy that yoga truly is for everyone, providing a safe, flexible, and inclusive path to health and wellness. This adaptability not only ensures that more people can participate in yoga but also helps them safely and effectively integrate these practices into their lives, promoting lasting health benefits.

CHAPTER 2

BREATHWORK AND MINDFULNESS: THE HEART OF CHAIR YOGA

"Change happens through movement, and movement heals."
[Joseph Pilates]

Breathwork and mindfulness are fundamental aspects of yoga that transform simple movements into powerful tools for enhancing physical and mental health. In chair yoga, these elements are emphasized to make the practice accessible and deeply beneficial, particularly for seniors or those with limited mobility.

Breathwork, or pranayama, involves controlling the breath to influence the flow of energy throughout the body. This practice is vital in chair yoga because it helps maximize the benefits of each pose by increasing oxygen intake and improving circulation. Controlled breathing also plays a crucial role in reducing stress levels and promoting relaxation. For instance, techniques like the diaphragmatic breathing encourage deep, full breaths that can help calm the nervous system and sharpen focus, making it easier to navigate the challenges of daily life.

In a chair yoga session, we might start by focusing on the breath before any physical movement begins. This helps to center the mind and prepare the body for exercise. Practicing breath control can significantly enhance the effectiveness of the yoga session, as it allows for a deeper connection between the body and mind, amplifying the benefits of the physical exercises that follow.

Mindfulness in chair yoga means being fully present in the moment, aware of one's body, thoughts, and feelings without judgment. This practice can be particularly transformative for seniors, as it encourages a greater awareness of the body's needs and limitations, fostering a gentler approach to movement and exercise. Mindfulness during yoga helps to cultivate a state of mental clarity and emotional peace, which can be carried into everyday life.

Mindfulness in chair yoga involves focusing on the sensations of each pose, observing the breath, and paying attention to thoughts or emotions as they arise during practice. This can be particularly helpful for those dealing with chronic pain or anxiety, as mindfulness helps to decrease emotional reactivity, increase patient tolerance to discomfort, and improve overall psychological flexibility.

Furthermore, the combination of breathwork and mindfulness in chair yoga creates a full health regimen that not only strengthens the body but also calms the mind and nurtures the spirit. These practices teach valuable skills that seniors can use to enhance their quality of life, manage stress, and maintain mental and emotional balance.

MASTERING PRANAYAMA: BREATH CONTROL FOR VITALITY

Pranayama involves various techniques that manage the breath to improve the flow of energy in the body. These techniques can range from simple deep breathing to more complex practices like the 'Kapalabhati' (skull shining breath) or 'Nadi Shodhana' (alternate nostril breathing). Each technique has unique benefits and can be adapted to fit the needs and capabilities of chair yoga participants.

Benefits of Pranayama in Chair Yoga

1. Enhanced Lung Capacity and Circulation: Regular practice of pranayama increases lung capacity and enhances blood circulation. Seniors can especially benefit from this because respiratory function tends to deteriorate with age.. Improved breathing not only supports better physical health but also ensures that vital organs receive the oxygen-rich blood they need to function effectively.

2. Stress Reduction: Breath control techniques are excellent for managing stress. By focusing on the breath, practitioners can shift their response to stress from a typical 'fight or flight' mode to a more relaxed 'rest and digest' state. This transition is facilitated by the parasympathetic nervous system, which helps to calm the body and mind, promoting a state of relaxation.

3. Boosted Energy Levels: Pranayama can also invigorate the body. Techniques like the 'Bhastrika' (bellows breath) are known for their energizing effects, which can be especially invigorating for individuals who spend much of their day seated or who have limited opportunities for physical activity.

4. Improved Mental Focus and Clarity: Regular practice of breath control helps to clear the mind, improve concentration, and enhance cognitive function. For seniors, this aspect of pranayama is invaluable as it contributes to better mental health and a sharper mind.

Integrating Pranayama into Chair Yoga Routines

Adding pranayama into a chair yoga routine is straightforward. A session might begin with a few minutes of focused breathing to center and calm participants before moving into more dynamic breathing exercises paired with gentle movements. Ending the session with a period of deep, meditative breathing can help consolidate the energy and peace cultivated during practice.

For those new to pranayama, it's important to start slowly and with guidance. Initially focusing on mastering the basics such as deep abdominal breathing sets a solid foundation. As confidence and comfort with these techniques grow, more advanced practices can be introduced gradually.

Mastering pranayama within the context of chair yoga not only enhances physical health and vitality but also brings profound benefits to mental and emotional well-being, making it a cornerstone of a holistic approach to senior health care. Through deliberate and mindful breath control, seniors can unlock remarkable improvements in their overall quality of life.

THE POWER OF NOW: CULTIVATING MINDFULNESS THROUGH MEDITATION

Meditation and mindfulness are key practices in yoga that focus on the present moment to allows a deeper sense of peace and awareness. In chair yoga, these practices are particularly beneficial as they enhance the mental and emotional aspects of health, helping participants to connect with the 'now'—the present moment where life's richness truly unfolds.

Understanding Mindfulness and Meditation

Being completely present and involved in the present, while remaining judgement- and distraction-free yet conscious of your thoughts and feelings, is the practice of mindfulness. Meditation, often used as a tool to enhance mindfulness, involves specific techniques to focus and quiet the mind, leading to greater mental clarity and emotional calm.

These practices offer profound benefits, particularly in a world where our attention is often fragmented by constant stimuli and distractions. For seniors, who may be dealing with various stressors such as health concerns or lifestyle changes, mindfulness and meditation provide essential tools for managing stress, reducing anxiety, and cultivating a more peaceful state of mind.

Mindfulness in Chair Yoga

Integrating mindfulness into chair yoga sessions is straightforward and enriching. A typical session might begin with a short meditation to center the mind and establish a connection to the present moment. Participants are encouraged to focus on their breath or a specific object of meditation, gently guiding their attention back whenever it wanders. This practice not only enhances the yoga session but also trains the mind to remain focused and serene throughout the day.

Throughout the yoga practice, mindfulness continues as participants are guided to pay attention to their body's sensations, thoughts, and emotions as they move through each pose. This ongoing awareness nurtures a deep connection between mind and body, enhancing the overall effectiveness of the exercises.

Benefits of Mindfulness Meditation in Chair Yoga

1. Stress Reduction: Regular mindfulness meditation significantly lowers stress levels by reducing the production of stress hormones such as cortisol. This calming effect can have wide-ranging health benefits, including lowering blood pressure and improving sleep patterns.

2. Enhanced Emotional Resilience: Engaging in mindfulness helps build emotional resilience, making it easier to handle life's ups and downs. This is crucial for maintaining mental health as we age, providing a way to process and respond to emotions more healthily.

3. Improved Cognitive Function: Meditation has been shown to improve attention, concentration, and overall cognitive function. These benefits are especially valuable for seniors, helping to counteract age-related declines in brain function and maintaining mental agility.

4. Greater Physical Health: While the focus of meditation is often on mental and emotional benefits, it also offers physical health advantages. These include reduced chronic pain, better immune function, and enhanced energy levels, all of which contribute to a more active and fulfilling life.

The Power of Now in chair yoga is about harnessing the benefits of meditation and mindfulness to transform not just moments of practice but all aspects of daily life. By cultivating a mindful approach, seniors can enjoy increased mental clarity, emotional peace, and a deeper appreciation of life's simple pleasures. This connection to the present is a powerful tool, leading to a richer, more fulfilling experience of life.

BREATHING AND MINDFULNESS AS A LIFESTYLE

Integrating breathing and mindfulness into daily life isn't just a practice; it's a lifestyle change that can significantly enhance one's quality of life, especially for seniors. These techniques are powerful tools in chair yoga, but their true potential is unlocked when practiced regularly in everyday activities, transforming ordinary moments into opportunities for growth and well-being.

Why Integrate Breathing and Mindfulness Daily?

Breathing techniques and mindfulness practices help manage stress, improve focus, and promote a balanced emotional state. For seniors, these benefits are particularly valuable as they navigate the challenges associated with aging. Regular practice can enhance physical health by improving respiratory efficiency, lowering blood pressure, and strengthening the immune system. Mentally, it sharpens cognition and fends off the cloudiness often associated with older age.

Practical Ways to performing Breathing and Mindfulness

1. Start the Day with Intention: Begin each morning with a few minutes of deep breathing and setting intentions for the day. This practice can help center thoughts and establish a calm, positive tone for the hours ahead.

2. Mindful Eating: Transform meal times into mindful practices by focusing on the flavors, textures, and sensations of eating. This not only enhances the enjoyment of food but also encourages better digestion and satisfaction with smaller portions, which is crucial for managing weight and digestive health.

3. Walking with Awareness: Turn regular walks into mindfulness exercises by concentrating on the movement of the body and the feeling of the ground under your feet. This not only increases physical activity but also connects you deeply with the present moment, enhancing mental clarity.

4. Breath Breaks: Incorporate short breathing exercises into the day, especially during moments of stress or tension. Techniques like the '4-7-8' breathing can be done almost anywhere and provide immediate stress relief and focus.

5. Mindful Listening: Engage in conversations fully by practicing mindful listening. This means listening to understand, not to respond, which improves relationships and deepens connections with others.

Mindfulness in Everyday Tasks: Bring a mindful approach to routine activities, such as gardening, washing dishes, or knitting. By focusing fully on the task at hand, you transform these ordinary activities into meditative practices that calm the mind and reduce feelings of anxiety.

The Benefits of a Mindfulness-Based Lifestyle

Adopting a lifestyle that emphasizes daily breathing and mindfulness practices offers extensive benefits. It leads to greater emotional balance, reduced stress, and a profound sense of presence and engagement with life. For seniors, this can mean not only better physical health but also a greater sense of purpose and joy in their daily lives.

With this, seniors can maximize the therapeutic effects of their chair yoga routines and enjoy a more serene, healthy, and mindful existence. This daily integration ensures that the benefits of chair yoga extend beyond the mat, influencing every part of the practitioner's life.

CHAPTER 3:

PREPARING FOR CHAIR YOGA: SETUP AND SAFETY

"A few well-designed movements, properly performed in a balanced sequence, are worth hours of sloppy calisthenics or forced contortion."
[Joseph Pilates]

Setting up properly and ensuring safety are critical when beginning a chair yoga practice, especially for seniors. A well-prepared environment and attention to safety can not only enhance the effectiveness of your practice but also prevent injuries and make the experience more enjoyable. Here's how to set up your space and prepare yourself for a safe and effective chair yoga session.

Choosing the Right Chair

The chair you use for your yoga practice is more than just a seat; it's an integral tool that supports your activity. Select a chair that is sturdy and stable, without wheels. The chair should have a firm, flat seat that isn't too soft, and it should support your back well. Ideally, when seated, your feet should rest flat on the floor, and your knees should be at a right angle. Avoid chairs with arms if possible, as they can restrict movement during certain poses.

Creating a Safe Space

Your practice area should be free from clutter and provide enough space for you to move your arms freely. Ensure the flooring around your chair is non-slip to prevent the chair from sliding. If you're on a particularly slick surface, place a non-slip yoga mat or a rug under the chair to secure it. Good lighting is important, too, so you can clearly see your surroundings and any guidance materials, like books or videos, you might be using.

Wearing Appropriate Clothing

Wear comfortable clothing that allows for movement but is not too loose, as baggy clothes can get in the way of poses or obscure your instructor's view of your alignment. Breathable, flexible fabrics work best to keep you comfortable throughout your session.

Setting Up Your Practice Area

If you like, you can enhance your practice area with elements that help create a calming atmosphere, such as soft music, dim lighting, or even a small indoor plant. These touches can help make your practice more enjoyable and relaxing.

SAFETY GUIDELINES

1. **Warm-Up:** Always start with a warm-up to gently prepare your body for exercise. This might include simple seated stretches or neck rolls, which help to loosen up the muscles and increase joint fluidity.

2. **Understand Your Body's Limits:** Be mindful of your body's capacities and any pain or discomfort you experience. Chair yoga is flexible and can be adapted to your needs. If a pose feels uncomfortable, try a modified version or skip it altogether.

3. **Stay Hydrated:** Keep water nearby and take breaks as needed to drink, especially if you're practicing longer sessions or feel tired.

4. **Use Props:** Don't hesitate to use props like cushions for extra support, straps to aid in stretches, or even a blanket under your feet if they don't reach the floor.

5. Practice Regularly: Consistency is key in any exercise regimen. Regular practice will help your body adapt to the movements of yoga and reduce the risk of strain.

By carefully preparing your space and respecting your body's limits, you can ensure a safe, enjoyable, and beneficial chair yoga practice. Remember, the goal of chair yoga is not just to perform every pose perfectly but to find balance, flexibility, and peace in a way that feels right for you.

SELECTING THE RIGHT EQUIPMENT

Choosing the appropriate equipment for chair yoga is crucial to ensure safety, comfort, and the effectiveness of your practice. While chair yoga requires minimal equipment compared to other forms of exercise, the right choices can significantly enhance your experience. Here's a guide to selecting the essential gear for your chair yoga sessions.

The Chair

The most important piece of equipment in chair yoga is, unsurprisingly, the chair itself. Here are key features to look for:

- Stability: Choose a chair that is sturdy and stable. It should not have wheels, as these can make it unstable and unsafe during exercises.
- Size and Height: The chair should be the right height for your body. When seated, your knees should be 90 degrees from the floor and your feet should be flat on the surface. This alignment helps maintain proper posture and prevents strain.
- No Arms: If possible, use a chair without arms, as this allows for greater freedom of movement during various poses and stretches.
- Material: A metal or wooden chair is typically more stable than plastic. Ensure the seat isn't too soft; a firmer seat provides better support during exercises.

Yoga Props

While not all chair yoga routines require props, having a few on hand can enhance your practice, especially if you have limited mobility or need additional support:

- Yoga Blocks: These can be used to support your hands, feet, or other parts of the body during poses, bringing the ground closer to you.
- Yoga Strap: A strap can help extend your reach and maintain alignment in poses where you need to hold onto your feet or legs.
- Cushions and Pillows: Use these for additional support under your feet, knees, or back, especially if you find certain poses uncomfortable or if the chair is too high.
- Non-Slip Mat: Placing a yoga mat or a non-slip pad under your chair can prevent it from sliding, especially if you are on a smooth surface.

Clothing

Comfortable, breathable clothing is essential for any form of yoga. Here's what to consider:

- Flexibility: Wear clothes that allow you to move freely but aren't too loose. Excess fabric can get in the way during poses.
- Fabric: Choose materials that wick away moisture and keep you comfortable throughout your practice.
- Layers: Especially if you are practicing in a cooler environment, wear layers that you can remove as you warm up during your session.

Additional Considerations

- Space: Ensure your practice area is spacious enough to move freely without hitting any obstacles.
- Personal Items: Have water nearby to stay hydrated, and consider a small towel to manage perspiration if needed.

By carefully selecting the right equipment for chair yoga, you not only make your practice safer but also more enjoyable and effective. Good equipment will help you maintain proper form, prevent injuries, and allow you to fully engage with your yoga practice, thus reaping the maximum benefits.

PERSONAL HEALTH ASSESSMENT AND TAILORING YOUR PRACTICE

Before diving into chair yoga, conducting a personal health assessment is crucial. This process helps you understand your current physical capabilities and limitations, ensuring that your yoga practice is safe, effective, and customized to your needs. Let's discuss how to assess your health and tailor your chair yoga practice accordingly.

Step 1: Evaluate Your Physical Health

- Consult with Healthcare Professionals: Before starting any new exercise program, it's advisable to consult with your doctor, especially if you have existing health conditions like heart disease, high blood pressure, or musculoskeletal issues. They can provide guidance on what exercises are safe and what to avoid.
- Assess Mobility and Flexibility: Note any areas of your body with restricted movement or pain. This will help you understand which areas need more attention and which poses to modify.
- Consider Your Balance: Evaluate how well you can maintain balance, as this will influence the types of poses you should focus on. Enhancing balance is a significant benefit of chair yoga, but starting with an understanding of your current level is important.
- Check Your Endurance: Reflect on how long you can engage in physical activity before feeling fatigued. This will help in planning the length and intensity of your sessions.

Step 2: Setting Your Yoga Practice

- Customize Poses: Based on your mobility, flexibility, and balance, adapt poses to meet your needs. Use props like blocks, cushions, or straps to help achieve poses comfortably and safely.
- Focus on Your Needs: If you have specific health concerns, like arthritis or back pain, focus on poses known to alleviate discomfort in these areas. For instance, gentle spinal twists can improve back health, while leg-strengthening poses can help with knee joint issues.
- Set Realistic Goals: Establish clear, achievable goals based on your assessment. Whether it's improving flexibility, building strength, or reducing stress, your goals will guide the focus of your sessions.
- Gradual Progression: Start with simple poses and short sessions. As your flexibility, balance, and endurance improve, gradually introduce more complex poses and longer practices.
- Monitor and Adjust: Continuously assess your progress and any changes in your physical condition. Be flexible in adjusting your practice to accommodate any new challenges or improvements.

Step 3: Engage Mindfully

- Listen to Your Body: Pay close attention to how your body feels during and after exercises. Avoid pushing into pain, and modify poses as needed to stay within a range of comfort.
- Incorporate Mindfulness and Breathing: Enhance the mental health benefits of your practice by integrating mindfulness and focused breathing techniques, which can help deepen relaxation and concentration.

Step 4: Seek Guidance When Needed

- Work with a Yoga Instructor: If possible, work with an instructor experienced in teaching chair yoga, especially when you're just starting out. They can provide personalized guidance and modifications to ensure your practice is safe and beneficial.

By taking the time to assess your health and tailor your chair yoga practice, you ensure a personalized approach that maximizes benefits and minimizes risks. This thoughtful preparation allows you to enjoy a more effective and rewarding yoga experience, tailored specifically to your health needs and wellness goals.

ESTABLISHING SAFETY PROTOCOLS FOR INJURY PREVENTION

Ensuring safety is paramount when practicing chair yoga, especially for seniors or individuals with mobility limitations. Establishing effective safety protocols can significantly reduce the risk of injuries and enhance the overall experience. Below is how to set up safety protocols for your chair yoga sessions.

Choose the Right Environment

- Stable Seating: Use a chair that is sturdy and stable without wheels. Chairs with a solid seat and back support are ideal. Ensure it does not wobble or tip when you move.
- Clear Space: Make sure your practice area is free from clutter and potential hazards. There should be enough space around the chair to move freely without bumping into furniture or other objects.
- Appropriate Flooring: Practice on a non-slip surface to prevent the chair from sliding. Place a yoga mat, rug, or non-slip pads under the chair and your feet for extra stability.

Proper Attire

- Clothing: Wear comfortable clothing that allows for movement but is not too loose to avoid catching or snagging. Opt for breathable fabrics to keep cool and maintain comfort.
- Footwear: Although yoga is typically practiced barefoot, non-slip socks or stable, flat shoes can be worn for additional grip and support if needed.

Personal Physical Preparedness

- Warm-Up: Always begin with a warm-up session to gently prepare your muscles and joints for exercise. This can include simple seated stretches or neck and shoulder rolls.
- Hydration: Keep water nearby and stay hydrated throughout your practice, especially in warmer conditions or during longer sessions.
- Know Your Limits: Be aware of your physical limitations and avoid pushing yourself too hard. Adapt poses and use props as needed to ensure comfort and prevent strain.

Instructor and Routine Considerations

- Qualified Instruction: If possible, work with a qualified yoga instructor who has experience with chair yoga and understands the needs of seniors or individuals with limited mobility.
- Routine Review: Regularly review and adjust your routine in response to your body's feedback. If a particular pose causes discomfort or is too challenging, modify it or consult with your instructor for alternatives.
- Feedback Mechanisms: Establish a system for ongoing feedback on your practice. Whether it's noting down how you feel after each session or discussing your progress with an instructor, feedback is crucial for adapting and improving your practice safely.

Emergency Preparedness

- Know How to Respond: Familiarize yourself with basic first aid and know what to do in case of an injury. Keep your phone within reach during practice to call for help if necessary.
- Inform Others: If you live alone, let someone know when you are practicing, so they can check in on you regularly.

Mental Preparation

- Mindfulness and Focus: Maintain a mindful approach to your practice, focusing on your movements and how they feel rather than on achieving the perfect pose. This mindfulness can prevent overexertion and help you enjoy the session more fully.

CHAPTER 4

SIMPLE WARM UP EXERCISES

"Every moment of our life can be the beginning of great things."
[Joseph Pilates]

SEATED MARCHING EXERCISE

Introduction

Seated Marching is an accessible and gentle exercise designed to promote cardiovascular health and strengthen the lower body, making it particularly beneficial for seniors. This exercise can be performed in the comfort of a chair, making it a safe option for maintaining fitness without strain.

Instructions

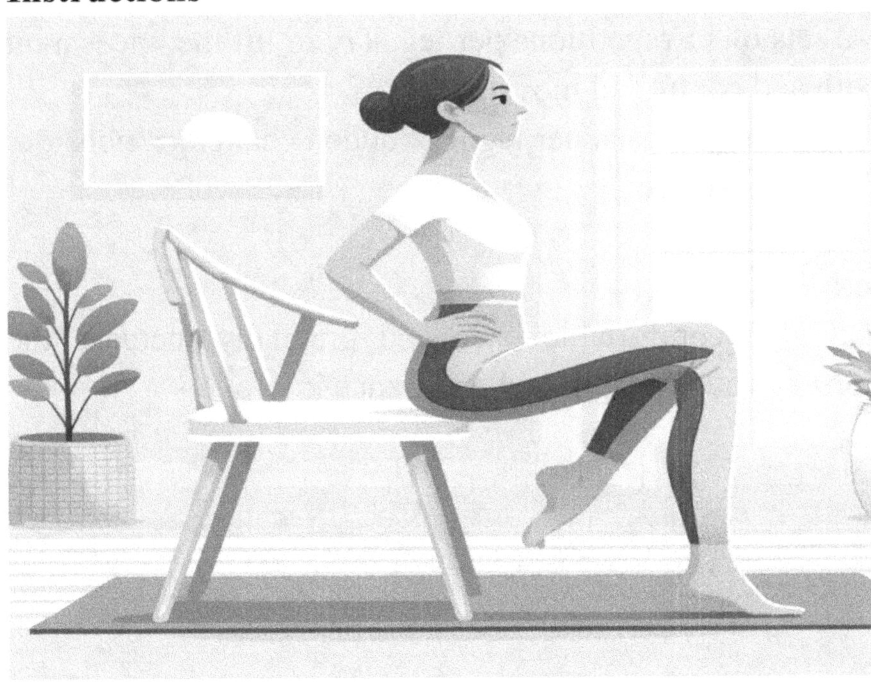

1. Starting Position: Sit in a sturdy chair with a straight back, feet flat on the floor, and hands resting on the thighs or by your sides.

2. Execution: Alternately lift your knees as high as comfortable, mimicking a marching motion. Keep the upper body stable and use your abdominal muscles to lift your legs.

3. Breathing: Coordinate your breathing by inhaling as you lift each knee and exhaling as you lower it, which helps engage your core and maintain rhythm.

Benefits

- Enhances Leg Strength: Strengthens the muscles in your thighs and lower legs.
- Improves Circulation: Increases blood flow and circulation through lower body movements.
- Boosts Cardiovascular Health: Helps raise your heart rate and improve heart health.
- Increases Joint Mobility: Promotes flexibility and movement in the hips and knees.

Routine for Different Skill Levels

- Beginners: Start with 1 set of 10 repetitions per leg. Focus on maintaining good posture and gentle movements.
- Intermediate: Increase to 2 sets of 15 repetitions per leg. Try to lift the knees a bit higher while ensuring smooth and controlled movements.
- Advanced: Perform 3 sets of 20 repetitions per leg. For added challenge, consider using ankle weights to increase resistance.

Number of Sets and Repetitions

- General Guidance: Begin at a comfortable pace and gradually increase the number of sets and repetitions as your strength and endurance improve.

ANKLE FLEX AND POINT EXERCISE

Introduction

The Ankle Flex and Point exercise is a simple yet effective way to improve flexibility and circulation in the lower legs, particularly around the ankles. This exercise is especially beneficial for seniors as it can help maintain mobility in the ankle joint, which is crucial for balance and walking.

Instructions

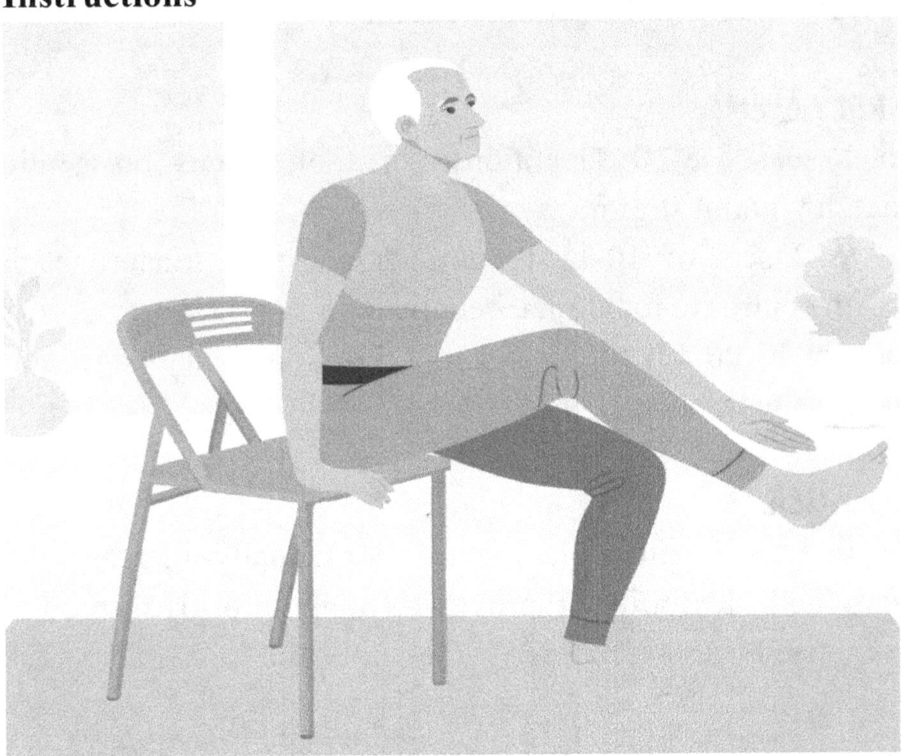

1. Starting Position: Sit upright in a sturdy chair without arms, ensuring your back is supported by the chair. Place your feet flat on the floor.

2. Execution: Extend one leg out in front of you with your foot off the floor. Slowly point your toes away from you, stretching the front of the ankle. Then, flex your toes back towards you, stretching the calf and the back of the ankle. Alternate between pointing and flexing smoothly.

3. Breathing: Inhale deeply as you flex your foot upwards, and exhale as you point your toes downwards. Proper breathing helps enhance the relaxation effect of the exercise.

Benefits
- Improves Blood Circulation: This exercise promotes blood flow to the feet and lower legs, which is particularly beneficial for those who are less active.
- Enhances Flexibility: Regularly performing this exercise can improve the flexibility of the ankle joints and muscles of the lower leg, reducing the risk of injuries.
- Reduces Swelling: For individuals who experience swelling in their feet and ankles, this exercise can help alleviate these symptoms.
- Supports Mobility: Maintaining ankle flexibility is essential for mobility and balance, contributing to safer walking and standing activities.

Routine for Different Skill Levels
- Beginners: Start with 1 set of 5-10 repetitions per foot. Focus on gentle movements to feel the stretch without strain.
- Intermediate: Increase to 2 sets of 10-15 repetitions per foot. Ensure each movement is performed with control to maximize benefits.
- Advanced: Perform 3 sets of 15-20 repetitions per foot. For added challenge, add a light ankle weight to increase resistance.

Number of Sets and Repetitions
- General Guidance: Begin at a comfortable level and gradually increase the intensity as your strength and flexibility improve. Always prioritize smooth, controlled movements over speed.

SIDE NECK STRETCH EXERCISE

Introduction
The Side Neck Stretch is a gentle exercise designed to release tension and improve flexibility in the neck muscles. This exercise is especially beneficial for seniors, as it helps alleviate stiffness and enhance mobility in the neck, which is essential for maintaining a good range of motion and comfort in daily activities.

Instructions

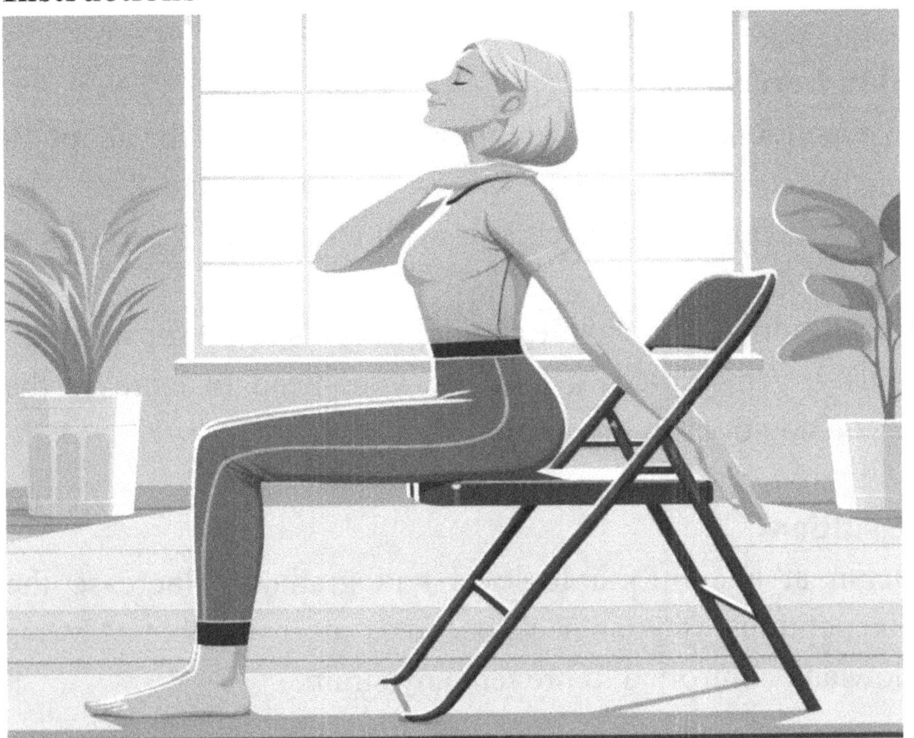

1. Starting Position: Sit upright in a sturdy chair without arms, feet flat on the floor, and hands resting gently on your lap.

2. Execution: Slowly tilt your head toward your right shoulder, aiming to bring your ear close to the shoulder without lifting the shoulder. Hold the stretch for a few seconds, feeling a gentle pull on the opposite side of your neck. Return to the starting position and repeat on the left side.

3. Breathing: Inhale deeply in the neutral position, and exhale as you tilt your head to the side. Keep your breath slow and steady to enhance relaxation during the stretch.

Benefits

- Reduces Neck Tension: Regularly performing this stretch can help relieve built-up tension in the neck muscles.

- Improves Flexibility: Increases flexibility in the cervical spine, which is vital for neck health and mobility.

- Enhances Blood Circulation: Stretching the neck muscles helps improve blood flow to the head and neck area.
- Decreases Headache Frequency: Can help reduce the frequency of tension headaches by relaxing the neck and shoulder muscles.

Routine for Different Skill Levels
- Beginners: Start with 3 repetitions on each side, holding the stretch for about 10 seconds each time.
- Intermediate: Increase to 5 repetitions on each side with a hold of 15 seconds to deepen the stretch.
- Advanced: Perform 7 repetitions on each side, holding each stretch for up to 20 seconds. For added intensity, gently place a hand on your head to increase the stretch slightly, ensuring you do not push too hard.

Number of Sets and Repetitions
- General Guidance: Begin at a comfortable level and gradually increase the duration and number of repetitions as your neck becomes more flexible. Always ensure movements are slow and controlled to prevent any strain.

WRIST AND FINGER STRETCH EXERCISE

Introduction
Wrist and Finger Stretches are essential exercises for maintaining the flexibility and strength of the hand joints and muscles. These stretches are particularly beneficial for seniors, as they help combat stiffness and pain associated with conditions like arthritis, and improve the dexterity needed for daily tasks.

Instructions

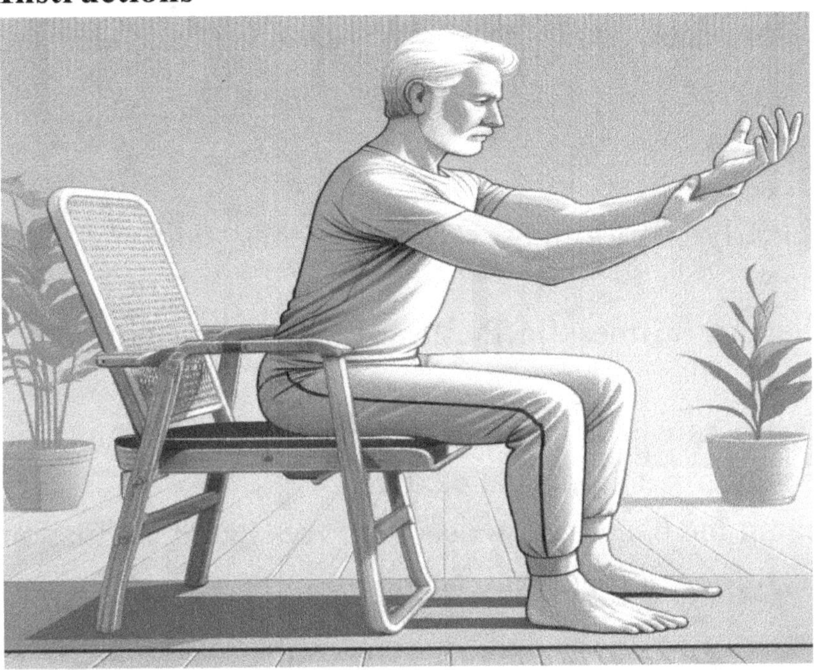

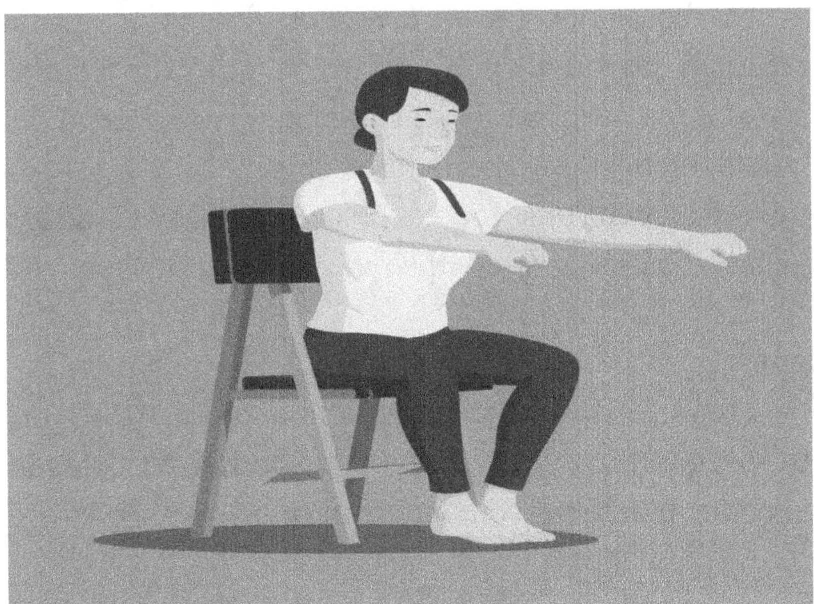

1. Starting Position: Sit in a sturdy, armless chair with your feet flat on the floor and back straight. Extend your arms forward at chest level.
2. Execution:

- Finger Stretches: Spread your fingers wide, hold for a few seconds, Then, slowly curl your fingers into a fist. Repeat several times to improve flexibility in your fingers.

- Wrist Stretches: Extend your arms forward and gently bend your wrists downward and then upward. Hold each position for a few seconds to stretch the wrist muscles and tendons.

Benefits

- Improves Flexibility: Regularly performing these stretches enhances the flexibility of the wrists and fingers.
- Reduces Stiffness: Helps alleviate stiffness in the hands and wrists, promoting smoother and pain-free movement.
- Increases Strength: These exercises can help strengthen the muscles around the wrists and hands, supporting better grip and manual dexterity.
- Enhances Circulation: Stretching the hands and wrists improves blood circulation to these areas, which is beneficial for cell repair and health.

Routine for Different Skill Levels

- Beginners: Start with 1 set of 5 repetitions for each stretch. Focus on gentle movements to ensure you do not strain the muscles.
- Intermediate: Increase to 2 sets of 8 repetitions for each stretch. Try to extend the range of motion slightly further, as long as it remains comfortable.
- Advanced: Perform 3 sets of 10 repetitions for each stretch. For an added challenge, you can use light resistance bands to strengthen the muscles further.

Number of Sets and Repetitions

- General Guidance: Begin at a comfortable level and gradually increase the number of sets and repetitions as your flexibility and strength improve. Always ensure movements are slow and controlled to prevent any strain.

SHOULDER CIRCLE EXERCISE

Introduction

Shoulder Circles are a gentle yet effective exercise aimed at enhancing shoulder mobility and relieving tension in the upper body. This exercise is particularly beneficial for seniors, as it helps maintain flexibility and reduce stiffness in the shoulder area, which is crucial for daily activities.

Instructions

1. Starting Position: Sit upright in a sturdy chair without arms. Feet should be flat on the floor, and your back should be straight but relaxed.

2. Execution: Lift your shoulders towards your ears, then gently roll them back, down, and then forward in a smooth circular motion. After completing several circles in one direction, switch and roll them in the opposite direction.

3. Breathing: Inhale deeply as you lift your shoulders up and exhale as you complete the circle down and forward. Proper breathing helps to increase the relaxation effect of the exercise.

Benefits

- Improves Flexibility and Mobility: Regularly performing shoulder circles helps increase the range of motion in your shoulders and upper back.
- Reduces Tension and Stiffness: This exercise is excellent for relieving tension and stiffness that often accumulates in the shoulder region.
- Enhances Circulation: Moving the shoulders in circular motions helps improve blood flow to the surrounding muscles.
- Supports Posture: By strengthening and loosening the shoulder muscles, this exercise can also contribute to better posture.

Routine for Different Skill Levels

- Beginners: Start with 1 set of 8-10 repetitions in each direction. Focus on performing the movements slowly and with control.

- Intermediate: Increase to 2 sets of 10-12 repetitions in each direction. Make sure every action is deliberate and fluid.
- Advanced: Perform 3 sets of 12-15 repetitions in each direction. Consider holding a light weight in each hand to increase resistance and strengthen the shoulder muscles further.

Number of Sets and Repetitions
- General Guidance: Begin with what feels comfortable, and gradually increase the number of repetitions and sets as your flexibility and strength improve.

CHAPTER 5:

FLEXIBILITY EXERCISES

CHAIR WARRIOR I

Introduction

Chair Warrior I is a modified version of the classic Warrior I pose, adapted for chair yoga to make it accessible and safe for seniors. This pose focuses on strengthening the legs, improving balance, and stretching the upper body, all while seated.

Instructions

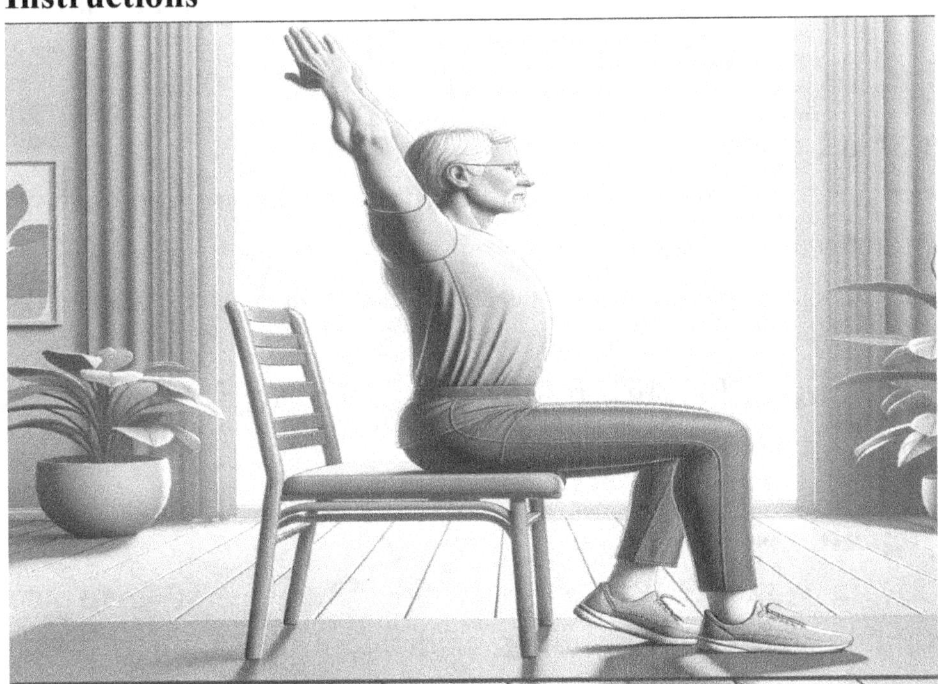

1. Starting Position: Sit on the edge of a sturdy, armless chair. Place your left foot flat on the floor, directly under your knee, and extend your right leg back, keeping it straight and the heel off the ground.

2. Execution: Inhale and raise your arms above your head, keeping them straight and your palms facing each other. As you settle into the pose, gently press your chest forward and up, maintaining a strong, straight back.

3. Hold and Breathe: Maintain this position for 20-30 seconds while breathing deeply. Feel the stretch in your right hip and leg and the engagement in your left thigh.

4. Switch Sides: Gently lower your arms and switch the position of your legs to repeat the pose on the opposite side.

Benefits

- Strengthens Lower Body: This pose helps strengthen the thighs and calves, improving overall leg strength.
- Enhances Balance: Regular practice can improve your balance, which is crucial for preventing falls.
- Stretches the Upper Body: Lifting the arms helps stretch the chest, shoulders, and arms, promoting flexibility.
- Boosts Focus and Stamina: Holding the pose enhances mental focus and builds endurance.

Routine for Different Skill Levels

- Beginners: Perform the pose with arms raised only halfway or keep them on your hips, focusing on leg strength and balance.
- Intermediate: Hold the full pose with arms overhead, increasing the duration to up to 45 seconds.
- Advanced: Intensify the stretch by pressing the chest more forward and arms further back, and hold for up to 60 seconds.

Number of Sets and Repetitions

- General Guidance: Begin with 1-2 sets on each side. As your strength and flexibility increase, you can add more repetitions or increase the duration of the hold.

CHAIR EXTENDED SIDE ANGLE

Introduction

The Chair Extended Side Angle is a modified version of the traditional Extended Side Angle pose, adapted for chair yoga to ensure it is accessible and safe for seniors. This pose helps to stretch the sides of the body and improve flexibility in the shoulders and legs, while also strengthening the muscles of the abdomen and legs.

Instructions

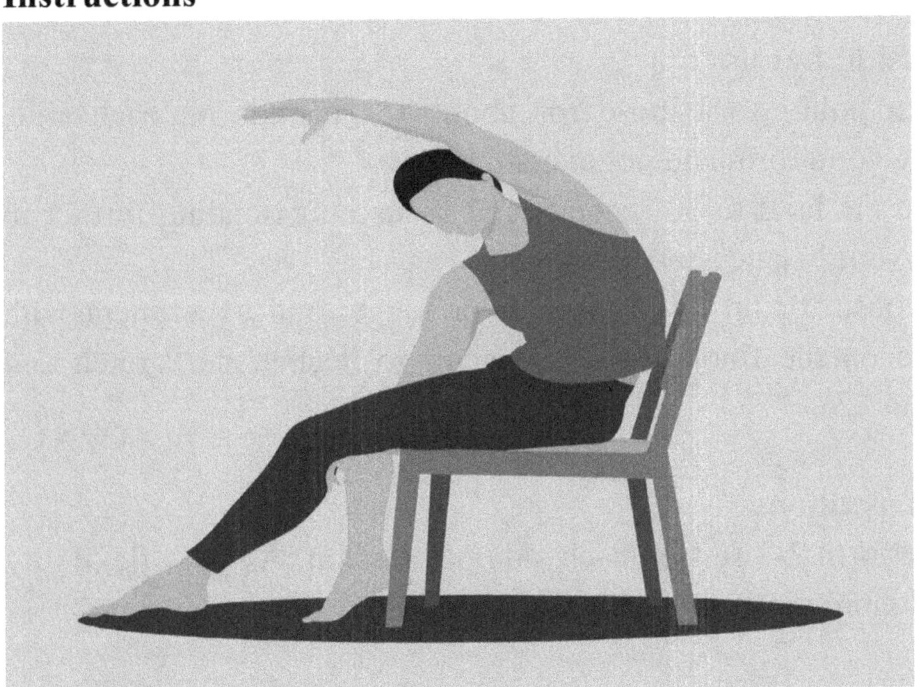

1. Starting Position: Sit on the edge of a sturdy, armless chair with your feet flat on the floor. Position your left foot slightly forward and keep your right foot back, so your legs are staggered.

2. Execution: Place your left hand on your left thigh. Inhale, and as you exhale, extend your right arm over your head, reaching towards the left side, while gently bending your torso over to the left. Keep your chest open and facing forward.

3. Hold and Breathe: Maintain this position for 20-30 seconds, breathing deeply and feeling the stretch along the right side of your body.

4. Switch Sides: Gently return to the starting position and repeat the exercise on the opposite side to ensure balance in your stretch.

Benefits
- Enhances Flexibility: This pose stretches the torso, shoulders, and thighs, enhancing flexibility and range of motion.
- Strengthens Core and Legs: Engaging the core and legs during the pose helps to strengthen these areas.
- Improves Posture: Regular practice of this pose can help improve posture and reduce discomfort in the back and shoulders.
- Promotes Respiratory Health: The expansive nature of the pose encourages deeper breathing, which is beneficial for respiratory health.

Routine for Different Skill Levels
- Beginners: Start with holding the pose for about 15 seconds on each side, focusing on maintaining good form and not overstretching.
- Intermediate: Increase the hold to 30 seconds and focus on extending further in the pose while keeping your balance and alignment.
- Advanced: Hold the pose for up to 45 seconds or longer and experiment with placing the lower hand on the floor beside the chair to deepen the stretch and increase the challenge.

Number of Sets and Repetitions
- General Guidance: Perform 2-3 sets on each side per session. As your flexibility increases, you may add more repetitions or hold the pose longer.

SEATED FORWARD BEND

Introduction
The Seated Forward Bend is a gentle, accessible exercise for seniors that stretches the spine and hamstrings while promoting relaxation. This pose is particularly beneficial for improving flexibility and can also help relieve stress and calm the mind.

Instructions

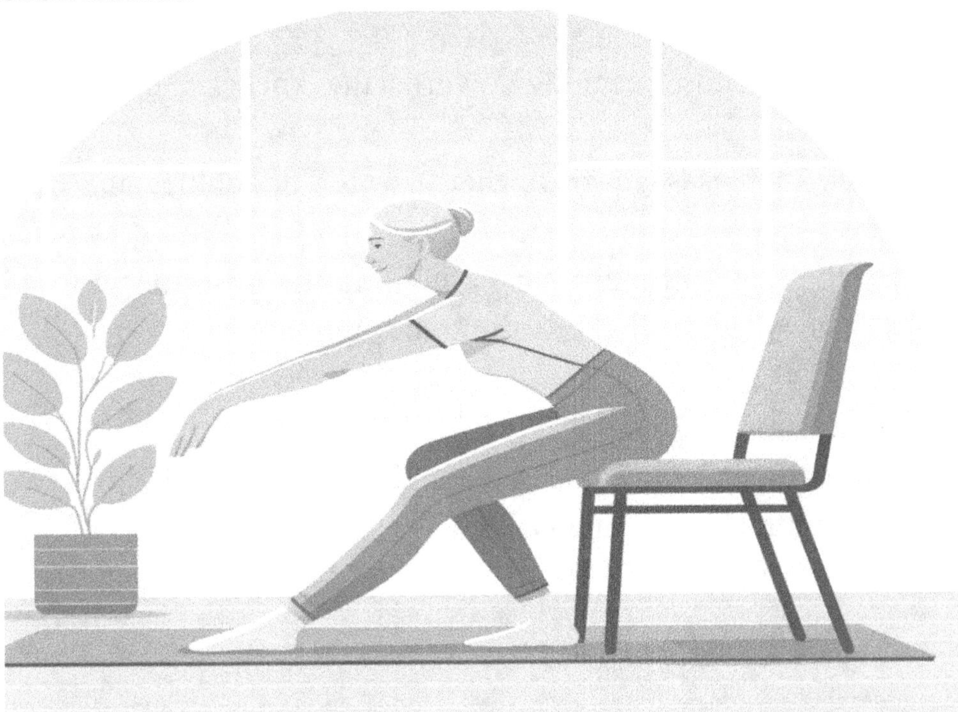

1. Starting Position: Sit at the edge of a sturdy, armless chair with your feet flat on the ground, hip-width apart.

2. Execution: Inhale deeply and, as you exhale, slowly bend forward from your hips, extending your hands towards your feet. Keep your back as flat as possible to avoid rounding the spine. Reach as far as comfortable, aiming to grasp your shins, ankles, or feet depending on your flexibility.

3. Breathing: Maintain deep, steady breaths throughout the stretch. Inhale as you prepare to bend, and exhale as you deepen into the forward bend.

4. Release: Gently come back up to the sitting position on an inhalation.

Benefits

- Enhances Flexibility: Regular practice of this pose can increase flexibility in the hamstrings and lower back.
- Promotes Spinal Health: The forward bend encourages a lengthening of the spine, which can help relieve compression and tension in the vertebral column.
- Reduces Stress: This pose has a calming effect on the mind and can help reduce anxiety and mental stress.
- Improves Digestion: The bending motion can stimulate abdominal organs, aiding in digestion and metabolism.

Routine for Different Skill Levels
- Beginners: Start with gentle bends, reaching towards the knees, and hold for about 10-15 seconds.
- Intermediate: As flexibility increases, reach further towards the ankles and hold the pose for 20-30 seconds.
- Advanced: Aim to grasp the feet with your hands, holding the pose for up to 45 seconds or longer, ensuring deep, controlled breathing throughout.

Number of Sets and Repetitions
- General Guidance: Begin with one set of the stretch and gradually work up to two to three sets as your comfort with the pose increases.

CHAIR PIGEON POSE

Introduction
The Chair Pigeon Pose is an adaptation of the traditional Pigeon Pose from floor-based yoga, making it accessible and beneficial for seniors or those with limited mobility. This pose focuses on stretching the hip rotators and the lower back, which can significantly enhance flexibility and reduce discomfort in these areas.

Instructions

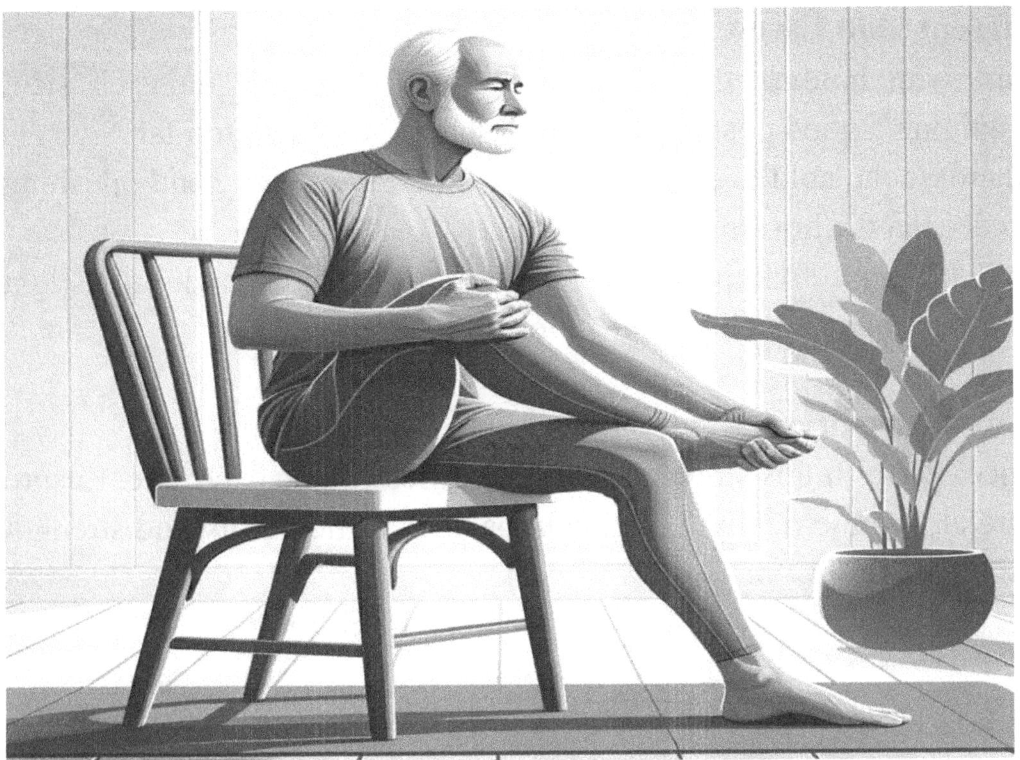

1. Starting Position: Sit upright in a sturdy chair without arms, feet flat on the floor.

2. Execution: Lift your right leg and place your right ankle on your left knee, forming a figure-four shape. Keep your back straight and gently press your right knee downwards to intensify the stretch. Ensure that you do not strain your knee joint.

3. Hold and Breathe: Maintain this position for 20-30 seconds while taking deep, relaxed breaths. Focus on releasing tension in your hip as you exhale.

4. Switch Sides: Gently release the stretch and repeat on the opposite side to ensure balance in the hip stretching.

Benefits

- Enhances Hip Flexibility: Regular practice improves flexibility in the hip joints and surrounding muscles, which can help prevent stiffness and maintain mobility.

- Reduces Lower Back Pain: By loosening the hip rotators, this pose can alleviate strain on the lower back, often reducing pain and discomfort.

- Improves Posture: Stretching the hip and lower back muscles can lead to better posture, reducing the likelihood of pain related to poor spinal alignment.

Routine for Different Skill Levels
- Beginners: Start with holding the pose for about 15 seconds on each side, focusing on maintaining a good posture without pushing the stretch too far.
- Intermediate: Increase the hold to 30 seconds and experiment with gently pushing the knee down to deepen the hip stretch.
- Advanced: Hold the pose for up to 45 seconds, and consider adding a slight forward lean to further engage the hips and lower back.

Number of Sets and Repetitions
- General Guidance: Perform this stretch 2-3 times per session on each side. Ensure to perform the stretch symmetrically to maintain balance in flexibility and strength across both hips.

CHAPTER 6:

CORE STRENGTHENING EXERCISE

CHAIR PELVIC TILTS

Introduction
Chair Pelvic Tilts are a gentle yet effective exercise aimed at strengthening the core muscles, specifically targeting the lower back and pelvic region. This exercise is particularly beneficial for seniors as it helps improve posture, reduce lower back pain, and enhance core stability.

Instructions

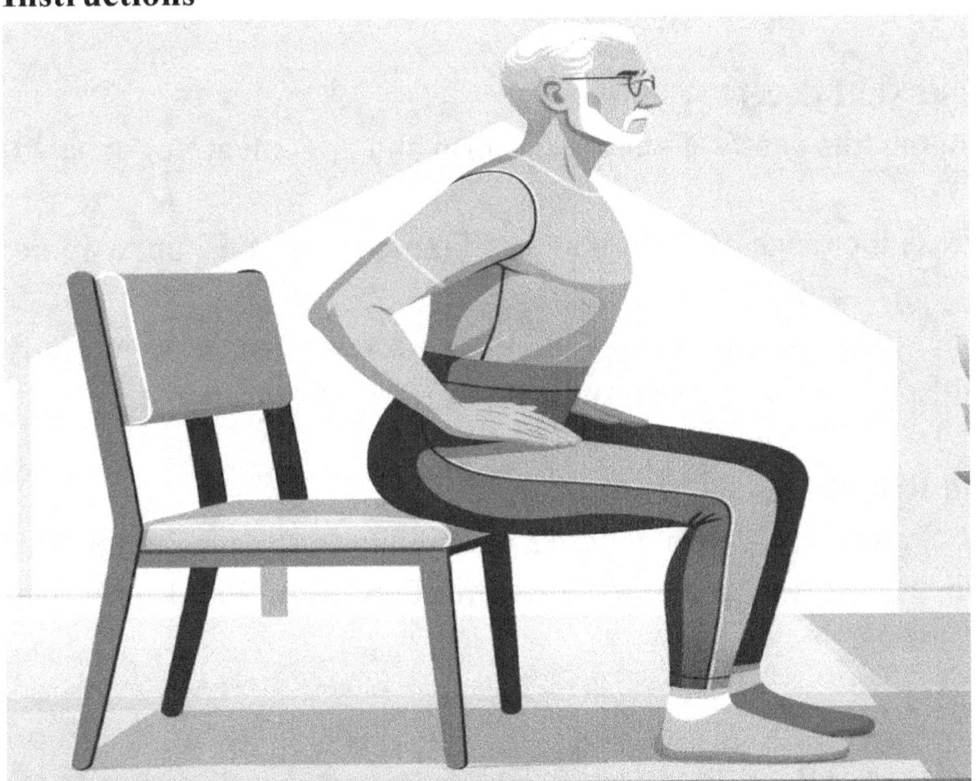

1. Starting Position: Sit upright on the edge of a sturdy, armless chair. Place your feet flat on the floor, spaced comfortably apart.

2. Execution: Place your hands on your hips or rest them on your thighs. Slowly arch your lower back and tilt your pelvis forward, then gently rock back to round your spine and tilt your pelvis backward. Ensure the movement is controlled and originates from your lower back.

3. Hold and Breathe: Breathe normally as you perform this tilting motion, focusing on smooth transitions and engaging your core muscles throughout the movement.

4. Repetition: Continue to tilt forward and backward for several repetitions.

Benefits

- Strengthens Core: Strengthens the muscles in the lower back and abdomen, crucial for overall stability and balance.
- Improves Posture: Regular practice can lead to better posture by aligning the spine and reducing the strain on the back.
- Reduces Lower Back Pain: Helps alleviate discomfort in the lower back through strengthening and mobilizing the pelvic area.
- Enhances Flexibility: Increases the flexibility of the lumbar region, promoting greater range of motion and mobility.

Routine for Different Skill Levels

- Beginners: Perform the tilts gently, focusing on form and alignment, for about 10 repetitions per set.
- Intermediate: Increase the range of motion and add more repetitions, up to 15 per set.
- Advanced: Integrate a hold at each end of the tilt for a few seconds to intensify the engagement of the core muscles, performing up to 20 repetitions per set.

Number of Sets and Repetitions

- General Guidance: Start with 1-2 sets of 10-12 repetitions and gradually increase as your strength and flexibility improve. Always prioritize control and form over the quantity of movements.

SEATED SIDE BENDS

Introduction

Seated Side Bends are an excellent exercise for enhancing spinal mobility and stretching the muscles of the torso and obliques. This gentle yet effective stretch is ideal for seniors as it can be performed while seated, making it safe and accessible for those with balance or mobility concerns.

Instructions

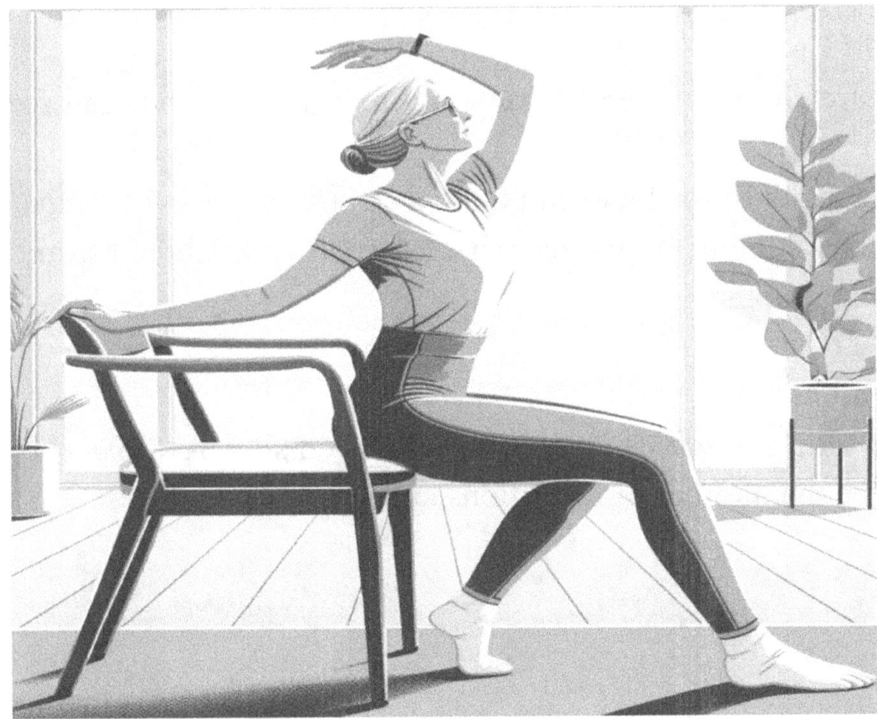

1. Starting Position: Sit upright in a sturdy chair. put your feet flat on the floor and hip-width apart
2. Execution: Place your right hand on the side or back of the chair for support. Inhale and extend your left arm straight up beside your ear. As you exhale, gently lean to the right, bending at the waist and extending your left arm over your head to deepen the stretch along your left side. Keep your hips firmly in the chair.

3. Hold and Breathe: Hold this position for a few deep breaths, aiming to stretch a little further with each exhale.
4. Return and Switch Sides: Slowly come back to the starting position on an inhale and repeat the stretch on the other side.

Benefits
- Improves Flexibility: Increases flexibility in the spine and lateral muscles of the torso.
- Enhances Respiratory Capacity: Opens up the ribcage, allowing for deeper breaths.
- Reduces Tension: Helps relieve tension in the shoulders and upper back.
- Promotes Spinal Health: Regular stretching of the torso can contribute to better spinal alignment and health.

Routine for Different Skill Levels
- Beginners: Perform the stretch with a gentle reach and less bending, holding for 3-5 breaths on each side.
- Intermediate: Increase the depth of the bend and hold each stretch for 5-7 breaths.
- Advanced: Try holding the stretch for longer periods, such as 10 breaths, and increase the frequency of repetitions.

Number of Sets and Repetitions
- General Guidance: Begin with 2-3 sets of 3 repetitions on each side. As flexibility improves, gradually increase the number of repetitions and sets.

CHAIR BOAT POSE

Introduction
The Chair Boat Pose is a modified version of the classic Boat Pose (Navasana), adapted for chair yoga to accommodate seniors or those with mobility limitations. This pose focuses on strengthening the core muscles, improving balance, and enhancing posture.

Instructions

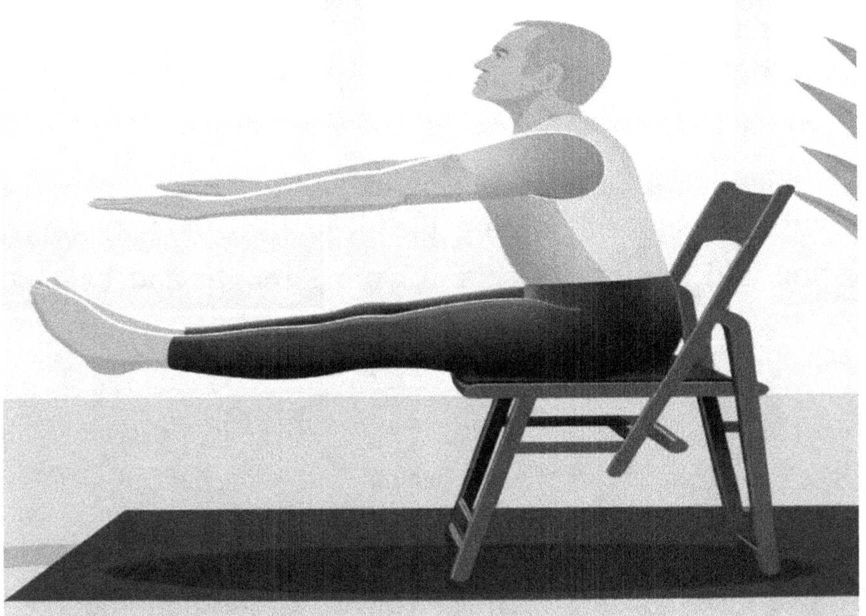

1. Starting Position: Sit at the edge of a sturdy, armless chair. Keep your spine straight and feet flat on the floor.
2. Execution: Lean slightly back without rounding your spine. Lift your feet off the floor, extending your legs forward. Simultaneously, extend your arms forward at shoulder height, parallel to the floor.
3. Hold and Breathe: Maintain this pose while taking deep breaths. Keep your core engaged and back straight. Hold the pose for as long as you can maintain good form.
4. Release: Gently lower your feet back to the ground and relax your arms.

Benefits
- Strengthens the Core: Engages and strengthens the abdominal muscles, which supports overall posture and back health.
- Improves Balance: Enhances your balance and stability, which is crucial for preventing falls.
- Increases Focus: Requires concentration to maintain balance and form, which can help improve mental focus.

Routine for Different Skill Levels

- Beginners: Keep your feet lightly touching the floor as you attempt to balance.
- Intermediate: Lift your feet higher off the floor and try to extend your legs more fully.
- Advanced: Hold the pose longer, aiming for up to 30-60 seconds, and work on fully extending the legs and keeping the arms parallel to the floor.

Number of Sets and Repetitions

- General Guidance: Start with 1-2 sets of holding the pose for 10-15 seconds. Gradually increase the duration and number of sets as your strength and balance improve.

SEATED KNEE TO CHEST

Introduction

The Seated Knee to Chest exercise is an effective way to strengthen the core muscles, improve lower back flexibility, and enhance abdominal control. This exercise is particularly beneficial for seniors as it can be performed safely while seated, making it accessible to those with balance or standing limitations.

Instructions

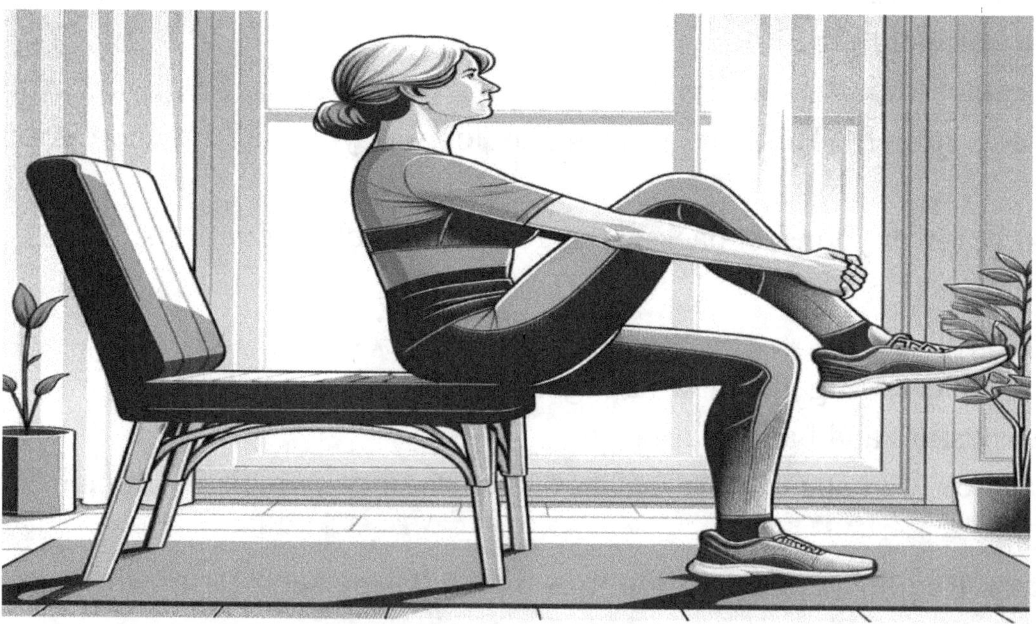

1. Starting Position: Sit upright in a sturdy chair without arms, feet flat on the floor.

2. Execution: Slowly lift your right knee towards your chest, using your hands to gently pull the knee closer while keeping your back straight. Ensure that you engage your abdominal muscles as you draw the knee in to maximize the core-strengthening benefits.

3. Hold and Breathe: Hold the knee against your chest for a few seconds while taking deep breaths. Feel the stretch in your lower back and the engagement in your abdominal muscles.

4. Release and Switch: Slowly lower your right leg back to the starting position and repeat the exercise with your left leg.

Benefits

- Strengthens Core Muscles: Regular practice helps strengthen the abdominals and lower back, supporting overall posture and balance.
- Improves Flexibility: This movement helps increase lower back flexibility, reducing the risk of back pain.
- Enhances Circulation: The motion increases blood flow to the lower extremities and the abdominal region.
- Promotes Digestive Health: The compression of the abdominal area can aid in digestion and alleviate bloating.

Routine for Different Skill Levels

- Beginners: Start with gentle lifts, focusing on maintaining balance and form, performing 5 repetitions per leg.
- Intermediate: Increase the hold at the top of each lift to 5-10 seconds, performing 8-10 repetitions per leg.
- Advanced: Add a light ankle weight to increase resistance, performing 10-12 repetitions per leg with longer holds.

Number of Sets and Repetitions

- General Guidance: Begin with 1-2 sets and gradually increase to 3 sets as your strength and endurance improve. Always ensure to perform the exercise symmetrically to maintain balance in muscle development.

CHAPTER 7:

MOBILITY EXERCISES

UPPER BODY MOBILITY EXERCISES

SHOULDER BLADE SQUEEZE

Introduction

The Shoulder Blade Squeeze is a simple yet effective exercise designed to strengthen the muscles around the shoulder blades, improve posture, and relieve tension in the upper back. This exercise is especially beneficial for seniors, as it aids in counteracting the common issue of rounded shoulders and promotes better spinal alignment.

Instructions

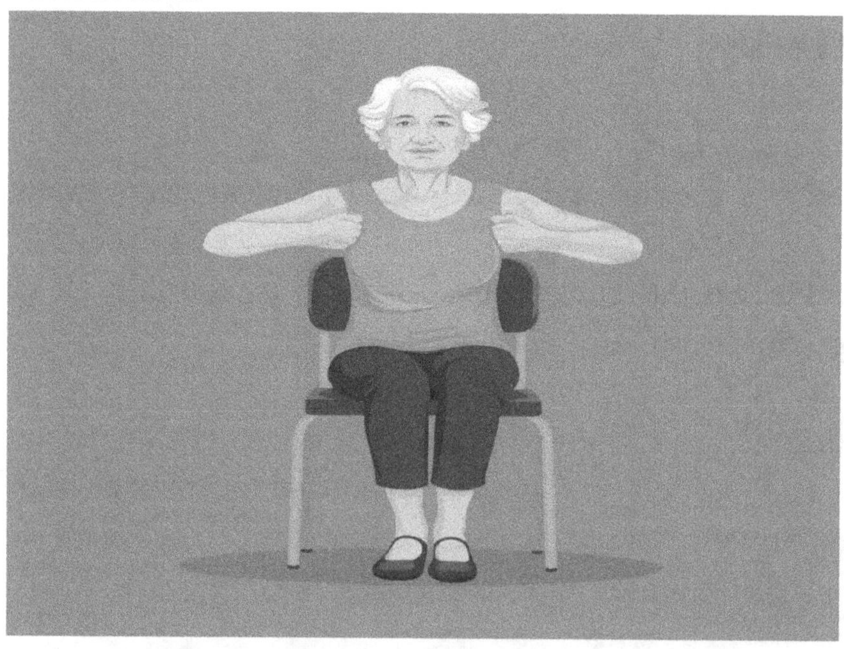

1. Starting Position: Sit upright in a chair without arms, feet flat on the floor, and hands resting on your thighs.
2. Execution: Inhale and gently pull your shoulders back, attempting to squeeze your shoulder blades together. Ensure the movement is controlled and focus on engaging the muscles in your upper back.
3. Hold and Breathe: Hold the squeeze for 3-5 seconds while maintaining normal breathing.
4. Release: Exhale and slowly relax your shoulders back to the starting position.

Benefits

- Improves Posture: Regular practice strengthens the upper back muscles, which are crucial for maintaining good posture.
- Reduces Tension: Helps alleviate tension and stiffness in the neck and shoulders.
- Enhances Mobility: Increases mobility in the shoulder region, making daily activities easier and more comfortable.
- Supports Spinal Health: Contributes to spinal health by promoting a more natural, upright alignment.

Routine for Different Skill Levels

- Beginners: Start with gentle squeezes, focusing on feeling the muscle engagement without straining. Perform 2 sets of 8 repetitions.
- Intermediate: Increase the hold time to 5-7 seconds and perform 3 sets of 10 repetitions.
- Advanced: Introduce variations by raising the arms to different positions to engage different parts of the upper back. Perform 3 sets of 12 repetitions with longer holds.

Number of Sets and Repetitions

- General Guidance: Begin with 2 sets of 8-10 repetitions and gradually increase the intensity and volume of the exercise as your strength improves.

SEATED CHEST OPENER

Introduction

The Seated Chest Opener is an excellent exercise designed to improve upper body posture and increase lung capacity. This stretch is particularly beneficial for seniors, helping to counteract the forward hunch often developed from prolonged sitting and everyday activities.

Instructions

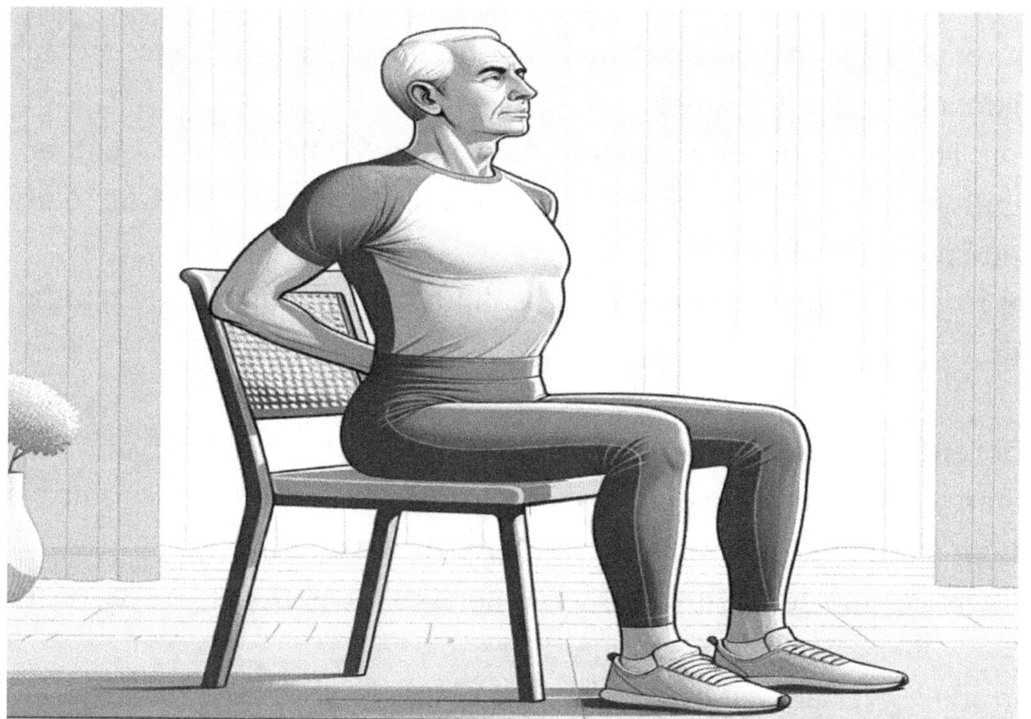

1. Starting Position: Sit upright in a sturdy, armless chair with your feet flat on the ground.

2. Execution: Place your hands behind your back, interlock your fingers, and gently pull your hands away from your back. Simultaneously, open your chest forward and lift your chin slightly, drawing your shoulder blades towards each other.

3. Hold and Breathe: Maintain this position for 15-30 seconds, taking deep breaths to help open your chest further.

4. Release: Carefully release your hands and relax your posture.

Benefits
- Enhances Postural Alignment: Regularly performing this stretch helps correct poor posture by strengthening the back muscles and opening the chest.
- Increases Respiratory Efficiency: By opening the chest, this exercise allows for deeper breaths, which can improve oxygen intake and overall respiratory health.
- Reduces Upper Body Tension: Alleviates tension in the shoulders and neck, common areas for stiffness.
- Promotes Flexibility: Increases flexibility in the shoulders and chest, essential for maintaining range of motion.

Routine for Different Skill Levels
- Beginners: Keep the stretch gentle, focusing on feeling a light stretch in the chest without discomfort.
- Intermediate: Increase the intensity of the stretch and the duration of the hold.
- Advanced: Intensify the stretch by clasping the hands tighter and pulling further, increasing the hold up to one minute.

Number of Sets and Repetitions
- General Guidance: Start with 2 sets of 3-5 repetitions each, gradually increasing the duration of the stretch and the number of sets as your flexibility and endurance improve.

OVERHEAD ARM CLASP

Introduction
The Overhead Arm Clasp is a straightforward and beneficial exercise aimed at enhancing shoulder flexibility and upper back strength. This movement is particularly useful for seniors, as it helps counteract the stiffness associated with aging and improves posture.

Instructions

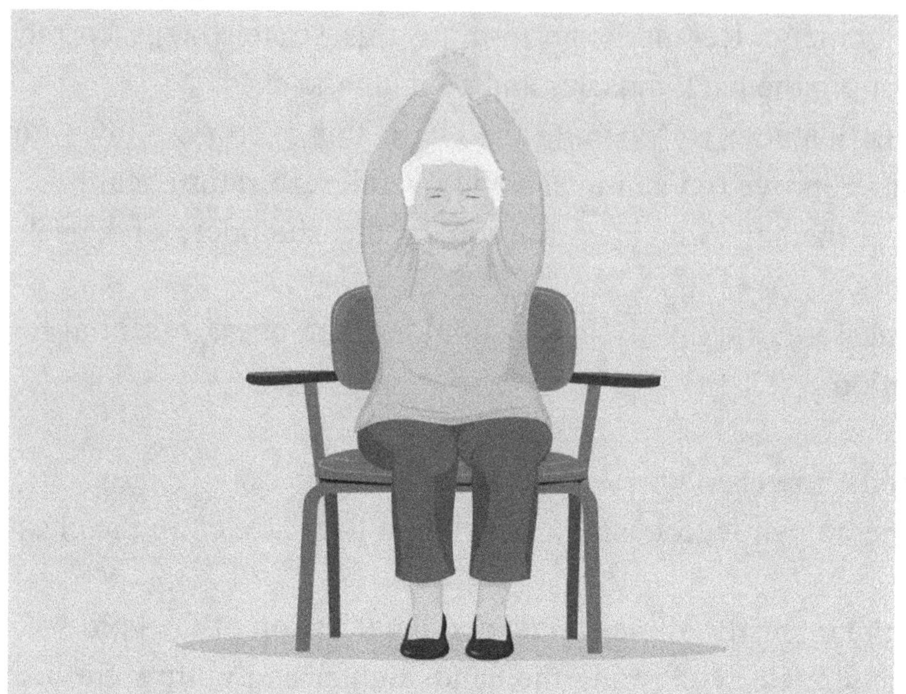

1. Starting Position: Sit upright in a sturdy, armless chair with your feet flat on the floor.

2. Execution: Raise your arms above your head and clasp your hands together, with your fingers interlocked. Gently pull upwards to feel a stretch in your arms and shoulders. Ensure your spine remains straight and you are not straining your neck.

3. Hold and Breathe: Hold this position for a few seconds while taking deep breaths, focusing on stretching further with each exhale.

4. Release: Slowly lower your arms and relax.

Benefits

- Improves Shoulder Flexibility: Helps increase the range of motion in your shoulders, reducing the risk of injuries.

- Strengthens Upper Back: Engages the muscles in the upper back, enhancing overall strength and posture.

- Alleviates Tension: Releases tension in the shoulders and neck area, often affected by poor posture or prolonged sitting.

- Promotes Better Posture: Regular practice contributes to a straighter, more aligned posture.

Routine for Different Skill Levels

- Beginners: Perform the exercise with less intensity, focusing on getting the form right without overstretching, for about 5-10 seconds per hold.
- Intermediate: Increase the duration of the hold to 15-20 seconds, ensuring smooth, controlled movements.
- Advanced: Aim to clasp your hands firmly and stretch more dynamically, holding for up to 30 seconds.

Number of Sets and Repetitions
- General Guidance: Start with 2-3 sets of 5 repetitions each, gradually increasing the number of repetitions and the intensity of the stretch as your flexibility improves.

SEATED CAT-COW STRETCH

Introduction
The Seated Cat-Cow Stretch is an essential exercise for improving spinal flexibility and relieving tension in the back. This gentle movement is particularly beneficial for seniors, helping to maintain a healthy posture and increase overall spinal awareness.

Instructions

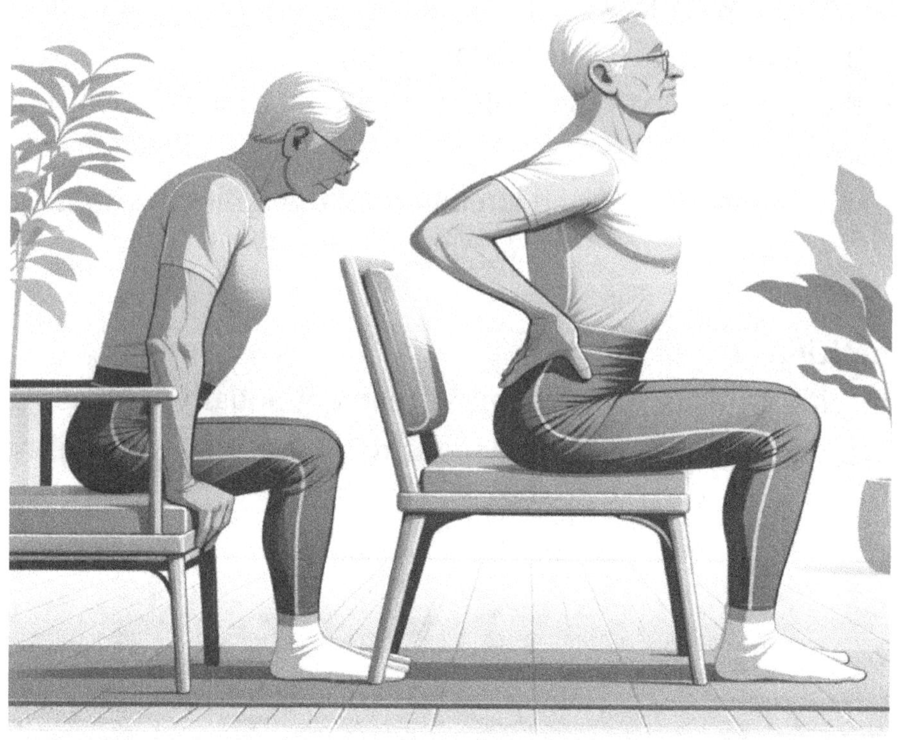

1. Starting Position: Sit on the edge of a sturdy, armless chair with your feet flat on the ground. Place your hands on your knees.
2. Cat Pose: As you exhale, round your spine, tuck your chin towards your chest, and draw your belly button towards your spine, creating a rounded back like a cat.
3. Cow Pose: As you inhale, arch your back, push your belly forward, lift your chin and chest, and look up, creating a cow-like curve in your back.you can put your hands on the side of the chair or back if comfortable.
4. Movement: Alternate between these two poses, moving smoothly with each breath.

Benefits
- Enhances Spinal Flexibility: Regularly performing this exercise can increase spinal mobility and ease stiffness.
- Reduces Back Pain: Helps alleviate back pain by strengthening and stretching the back muscles.
- Improves Posture: Encourages proper alignment of the spine and strengthens the core, which is essential for good posture.
- Promotes Relaxation: The rhythmic movement combined with deep breathing can have a calming effect on the mind and body.

Routine for Different Skill Levels
- Beginners: Focus on gentle movements, performing 3-5 repetitions of each pose.
- Intermediate: Increase the range of motion and hold each pose for a few seconds longer, performing up to 10 repetitions.
- Advanced: Integrate deeper stretches and longer holds, performing up to 15 repetitions or more.

Number of Sets and Repetitions
- General Guidance: Start with one set of 8-10 repetitions and gradually increase the number of sets and repetitions as your flexibility improves. Always ensure movements are slow and controlled.

LOWER BODY MOBILITY EXERCISES

SEATED HIP MARCHING

Introduction
Seated Hip Marching is a low-impact exercise designed to strengthen the hip flexors and improve mobility in the lower body. This exercise is especially beneficial for seniors, helping to enhance flexibility and balance, which are crucial for maintaining mobility and preventing falls.

Instructions

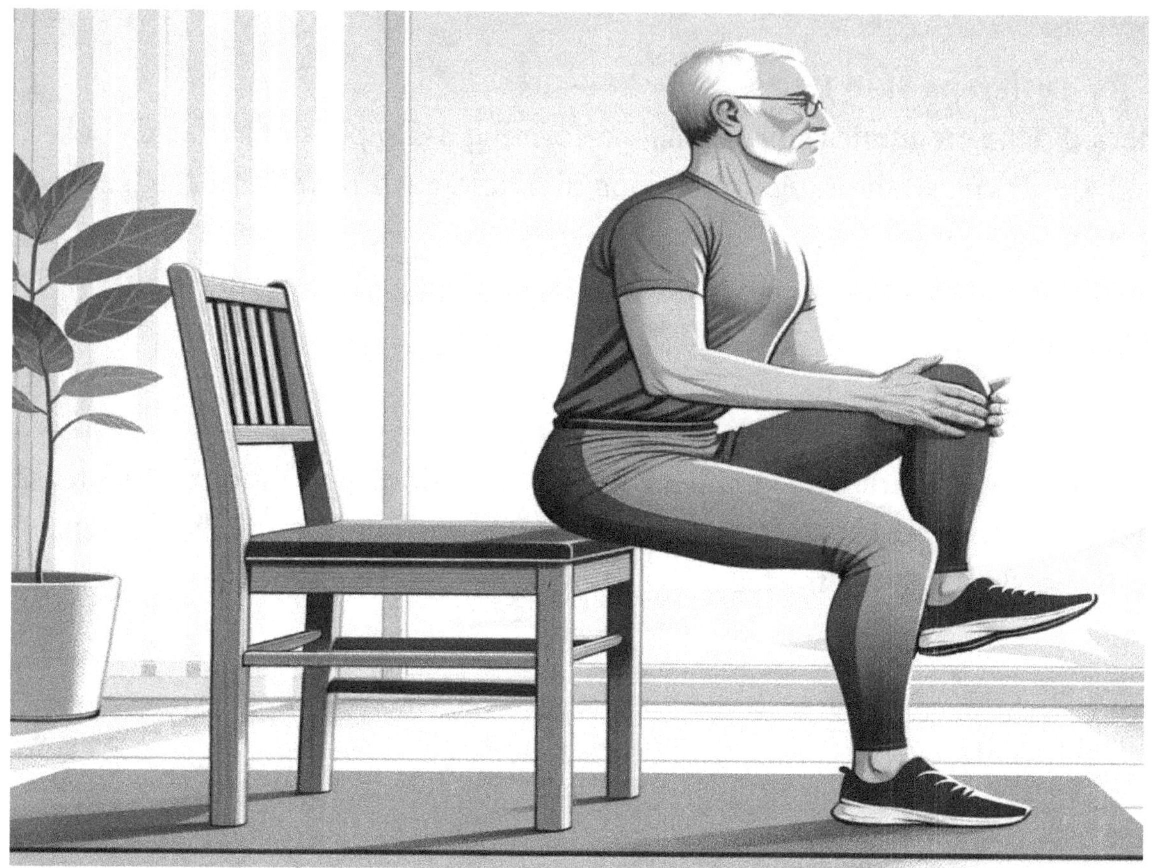

1. Starting Position: Sit upright on a sturdy, armless chair. put your feet flat on the floor and hip-width apart

2. Execution: Lift one knee toward your chest as high as comfortably possible, keeping the other foot firmly on the ground. You can use your hand to hold your knee for support. Hold the position briefly, then slowly lower your knee back to the starting position. Alternate legs with each repetition.

3. Breathing: Inhale as you lift your knee, and exhale as you lower it back to the starting position.

Benefits

- Strengthens Hip Flexors: Regular practice helps strengthen the muscles around the hips, supporting overall hip health.
- Improves Joint Mobility: Enhances the range of motion in the hip joints, which is vital for daily activities such as walking and climbing stairs.
- Promotes Circulation: Movement of the legs helps increase blood flow to the lower extremities, promoting better leg health.

- Enhances Balance and Coordination: By strengthening the hips and core, this exercise aids in improving balance and coordination, reducing the risk of falls.

Routine for Different Skill Levels
- Beginners: Perform the exercise slowly, focusing on maintaining balance. Start with 5 repetitions per leg for 2 sets.
- Intermediate: Increase the number of repetitions to 10 per leg for 3 sets. Focus on lifting the knee higher to increase the intensity.
- Advanced: Add a light ankle weight to increase resistance, performing up to 15 repetitions per leg for 3 or more sets.

Number of Sets and Repetitions
- General Guidance: Start with 2 sets of 5-10 repetitions per leg and gradually increase as your strength and flexibility improve. Ensure each movement is performed with control to maximize benefits.

SEATED LEG EXTENSIONS

Introduction
Seated Leg Extensions are a straightforward exercise tailored to strengthen the quadriceps muscles of the upper leg. This exercise is especially beneficial for seniors, promoting knee stability and overall leg strength, which are vital for daily mobility tasks.

Instructions

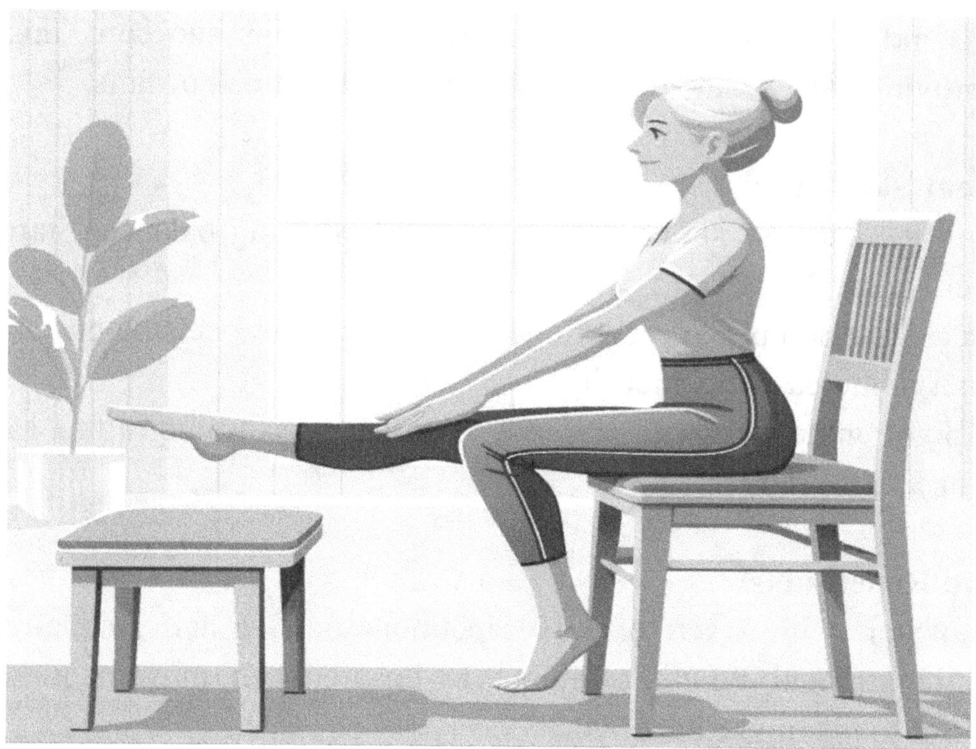

1. Starting Position: Sit upright in a sturdy, armless chair with both feet flat on the floor.

2. Execution: Slowly extend one leg in front of you until it is parallel to the floor. Keep your foot flexed and your back straight. Hold the leg extended for a few seconds.

3. Return: Slowly lower the leg back to the starting position.

4. Switch Legs: Repeat the exercise with the opposite leg.

Benefits

- Strengthens Quadriceps: Targets and strengthens the quadriceps, which are key for walking, standing, and maintaining balance.

- Improves Knee Health: Enhances knee joint stability and can help reduce the risk of knee injuries.

- Increases Flexibility: Promotes greater flexibility in the knee and hip joints.

- Enhances Circulation: Helps boost blood flow to the lower limbs, which is important for overall leg health.

Routine for Different Skill Levels

- Beginners: Perform the extensions slowly, focusing on form and control. Start with 2 sets of 8 repetitions per leg.

- Intermediate: Increase the hold at the top of each extension to 3-5 seconds and perform 3 sets of 10 repetitions per leg.
- Advanced: Add a light ankle weight to increase resistance, performing 3-4 sets of 12 repetitions per leg.

Number of Sets and Repetitions
- General Guidance: Begin with fewer repetitions and sets, gradually increasing as strength and endurance improve. Always ensure movements are smooth and controlled.

ANKLE ROTATIONS

Introduction
Ankle Rotations are a simple and effective exercise aimed at improving ankle mobility and flexibility. This exercise is particularly beneficial for seniors as it helps maintain joint function and can reduce the risk of falls by improving balance and coordination.

Instructions

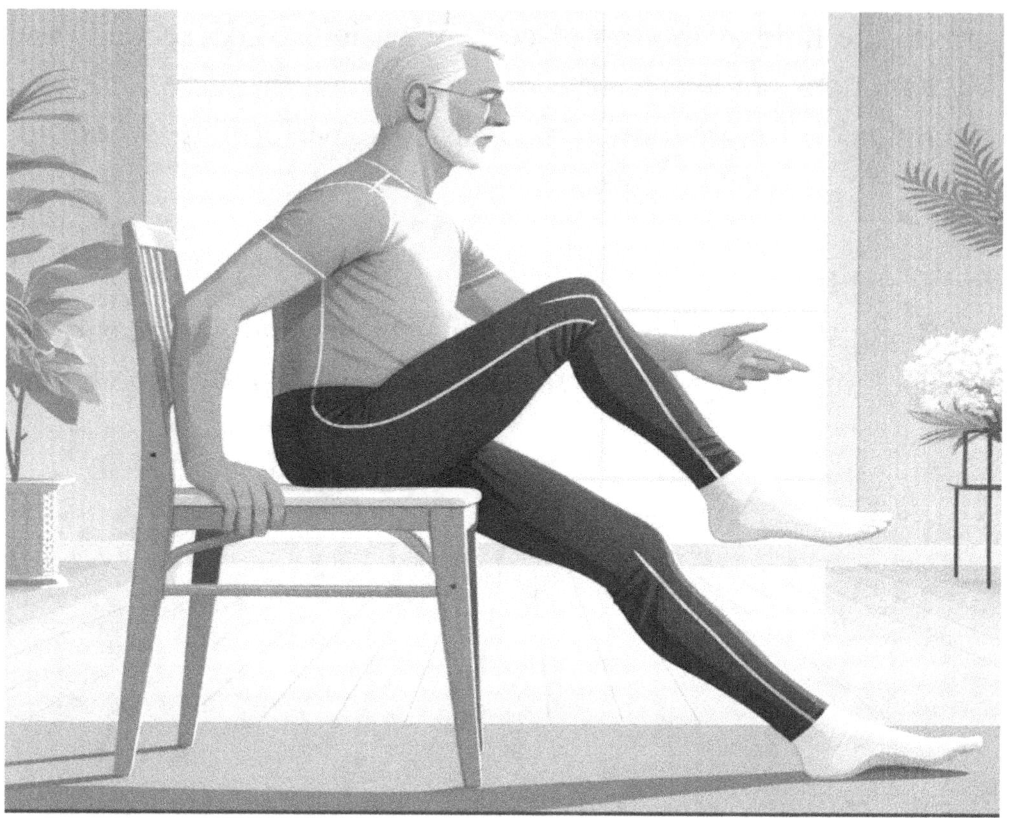

1. Starting Position: Sit upright in a chair without arms, with both feet flat on the floor.

2. Execution: Lift one foot off the floor. Slowly rotate your ankle clockwise for several rotations, then switch and rotate counterclockwise. Ensure the movement is controlled and originates from the ankle.

3. Switch Feet: After completing rotations with one ankle, lower the foot to the floor and repeat the same number of rotations with the other ankle.

Benefits

- Improves Flexibility: Regular ankle rotations increase flexibility in the ankles, aiding in smoother and safer movements.
- Enhances Circulation: These movements help enhance blood circulation in the lower extremities, which is beneficial for overall leg health.
- Reduces Stiffness: Helps alleviate stiffness and prevent ankle injuries by keeping the joints mobile.
- Supports Balance: Strong, flexible ankles are crucial for maintaining balance, especially in older adults.

Routine for Different Skill Levels
- Beginners: Focus on performing slow, controlled rotations, about 5 in each direction per ankle. Aim for 2 sets.
- Intermediate: Increase the number of rotations to 10 in each direction and add more sets.
- Advanced: Perform the rotations with a slight resistance band around the foot for increased difficulty, aiming for multiple sets of 10 rotations in each direction.

Number of Sets and Repetitions
- General Guidance: Start with 2 sets of 5 rotations in each direction per ankle. Gradually increase the number of rotations and sets as your ankle strength and flexibility improve.

CHAPTER 8:

STABILITY AND POSTURE EXERCISES

SEATED CHAIR BRIDGE POSE

Introduction

The Seated Chair Bridge Pose is a modified version of the traditional bridge pose, adapted for a chair to make it accessible for seniors or individuals with limited mobility. This exercise focuses on strengthening the lower back, glutes, and hamstrings while seated.

Instructions

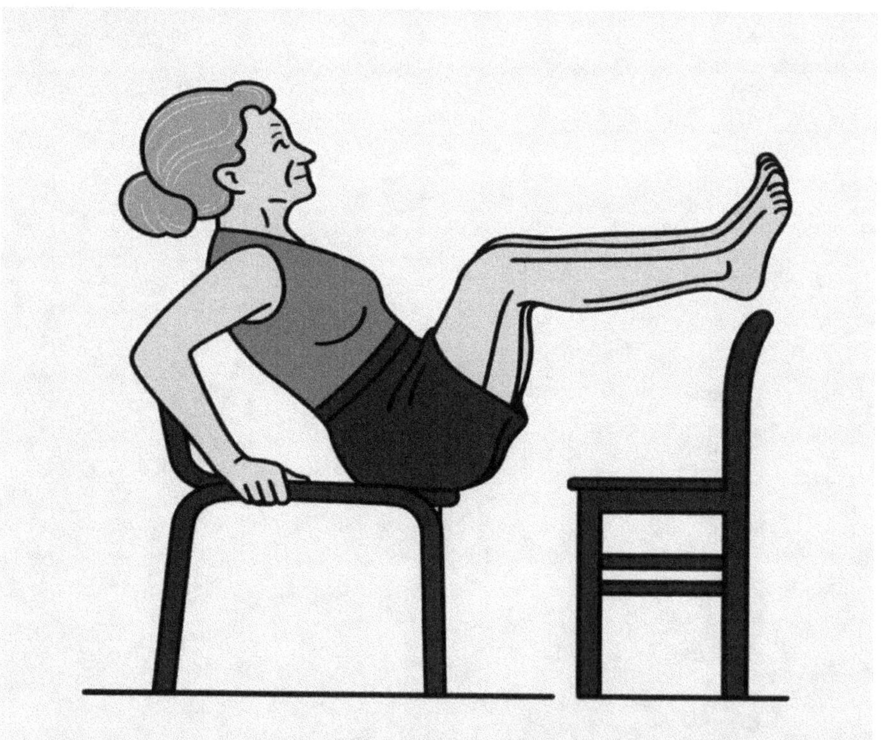

1. Starting Position: Sit near the edge of a sturdy, armless chair with your feet flat on the floor and knees bent.

2. Execution: Place your hands on the seat of the chair behind you for support. Lean back slightly and lift your hips upward towards the ceiling, trying to create a straight line from your knees to your shoulders. Engage your core and glutes to maintain stability.

3. Hold and Breathe: Hold this position for a few seconds while breathing deeply.

4. Release: Gently lower your hips back to the seated position.

Benefits
- Strengthens Lower Back and Glutes: Targets the muscles in the lower back and buttocks, enhancing strength and endurance.
- Improves Core Stability: Engages the abdominal muscles, promoting better core stability and balance.
- Reduces Lower Back Pain: Can help alleviate discomfort in the lower back through strengthening and gentle stretching.
- Increases Circulation: Promotes increased blood flow to the lower extremities.

Routine for Different Skill Levels
- Beginners: Perform the pose with a mild lift, focusing on form and comfort. Start with 2 sets of 5 repetitions.
- Intermediate: Increase the height of the hip lift and hold the pose for a longer duration, up to 10 seconds. Aim for 3 sets of 8 repetitions.
- Advanced: Add a small weight on the lap for added resistance, performing 3 sets of 10 repetitions with longer holds.

Number of Sets and Repetitions
- General Guidance: Begin with lower intensity and fewer repetitions. Gradually increase the duration of the hold and the number of sets as your strength improves.

CHAIR ASSISTED TRIANGLE POSE

Introduction

The Chair Assisted Triangle Pose is a gentle adaptation of the classic Triangle Pose, using a chair to make it accessible and safe for seniors. This pose helps stretch and strengthen the legs, improves flexibility in the hips and spine, and enhances overall balance and stability.

Instructions

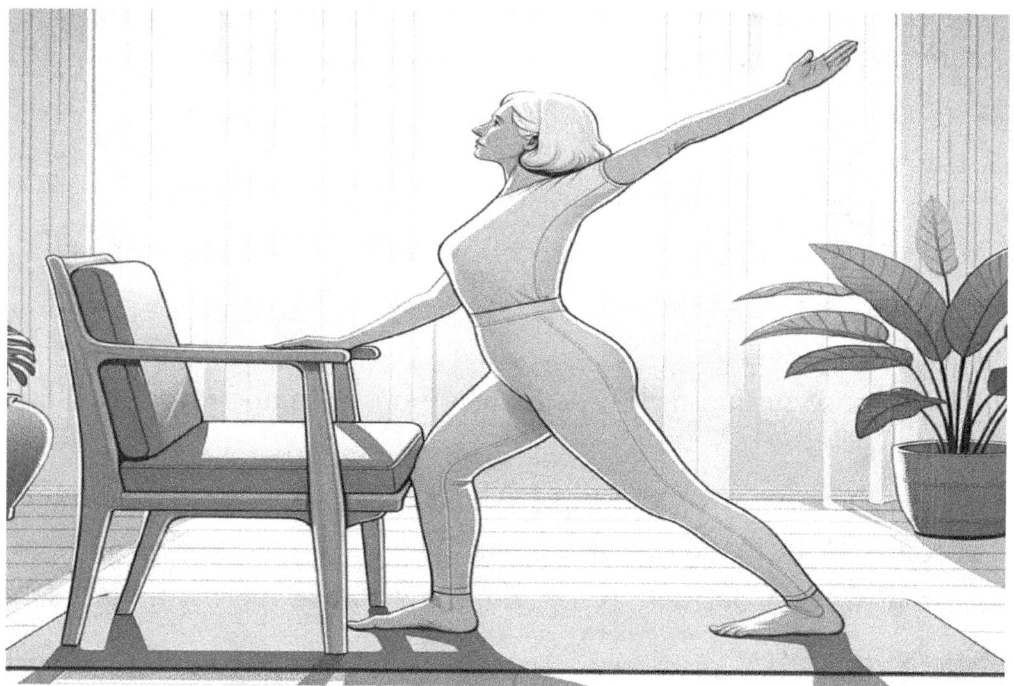

1. Starting Position: Stand next to a chair, placing it in front of you. Step your feet wide apart, approximately the length of one leg.
2. Execution: Turn your right foot out 90 degrees and your left foot in slightly. Extend your arms to the sides at shoulder height. Place your right hand on the seat of the chair for support. Stretch your left arm upwards, keeping your shoulders stacked and your gaze towards your left hand.
3. Hold and Breathe: Maintain this position, ensuring your body is stretched and open. Hold the pose for 15-30 seconds while breathing deeply.
4. Release and Switch Sides: Return to the starting position and switch the chair to the other side to repeat the pose.

Benefits
- Enhances Leg Strength: Strengthens the thighs, knees, and ankles.
- Improves Flexibility: Increases flexibility in the hips, groin, and hamstrings.
- Stimulates Abdominal Organs: Aids in the digestion and function of abdominal organs.
- Promotes Balance and Stability: Enhances proprioception and coordination, important for fall prevention.

Routine for Different Skill Levels
- Beginners: Use the chair for support and focus on maintaining balance with less deep stretching.
- Intermediate: Attempt to hold the pose longer, gradually decreasing the amount of support used from the chair.
- Advanced: Increase the duration of the pose and practice transitioning into and out of the pose smoothly without chair support.

Number of Sets and Repetitions
- General Guidance: Begin with 2 sets of the pose on each side, holding each for 15-30 seconds. Gradually increase the duration and intensity as flexibility and strength improve.

CHAIR PLANK POSE

Introduction
The Chair Plank Pose is a modified version of the traditional plank pose, adapted to be performed using a chair. This adaptation makes it more accessible for seniors or those with limited mobility, focusing on strengthening the core, arms, and shoulders while improving overall stability.

Instructions

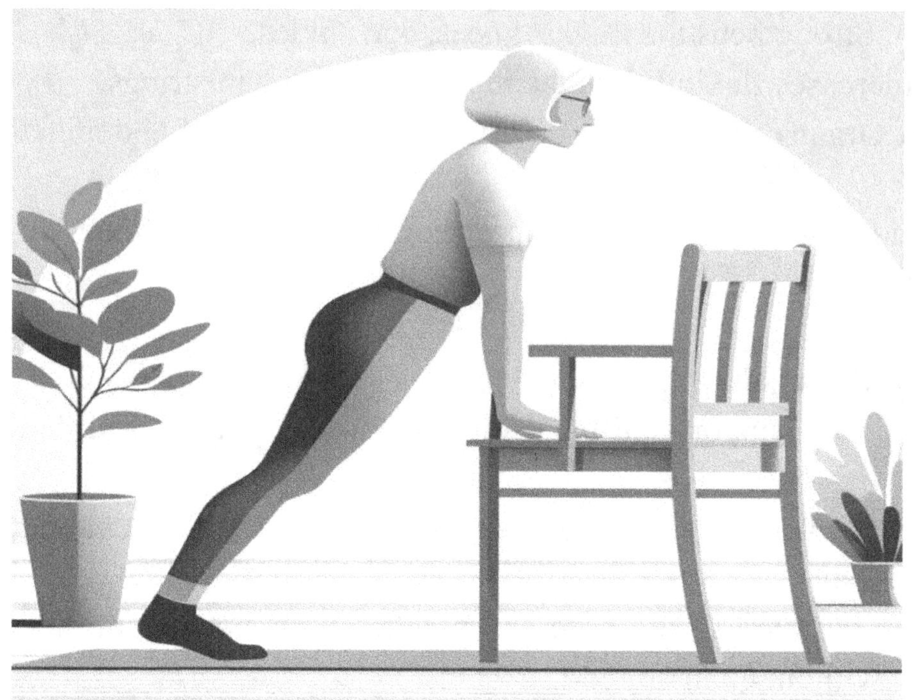

1. Starting Position: Stand in front of a sturdy, armless chair. Place your hands on the seat of the chair, shoulder-width apart.
2. Execution: Step your feet back until your body forms a straight line from your head to your heels, like a plank. Keep your hands firmly on the chair, and your feet planted on the ground. Ensure your core is engaged, and your back is straight.
3. Hold and Breathe: Maintain this position, keeping your body as straight as possible. Focus on breathing deeply to maintain the pose without sagging your hips or arching your back.
4. Release: Gently step forward to return to a standing position and relax.

Benefits

- Strengthens Core Muscles: Engages and strengthens the abdominal and lower back muscles, crucial for good posture and balance.
- Improves Upper Body Strength: Enhances strength in the shoulders, arms, and chest.
- Increases Stability: Helps improve balance and stability, reducing the risk of falls.
- Enhances Postural Alignment: Promotes a stronger, more aligned posture through core engagement and back strengthening.

Routine for Different Skill Levels

- Beginners: Hold the plank for 10-15 seconds, performing 2-3 sets.
- Intermediate: Increase the hold to 20-30 seconds and perform 3-4 sets.
- Advanced: Aim to hold the plank for up to 45-60 seconds, adding variations such as lifting one leg slightly off the ground for extra challenge.

Number of Sets and Repetitions

- General Guidance: Begin with shorter holds and fewer sets. As your strength and endurance improve, gradually increase both the duration of the hold and the number of sets.

SEATED SPINAL TWIST WITH ARM REACH

Introduction

The Seated Spinal Twist with Arm Reach is a dynamic exercise designed to enhance spinal mobility, flexibility, and overall core strength. This exercise is particularly beneficial for seniors as it helps improve posture, alleviate back pain, and increase overall spinal health.

Instructions

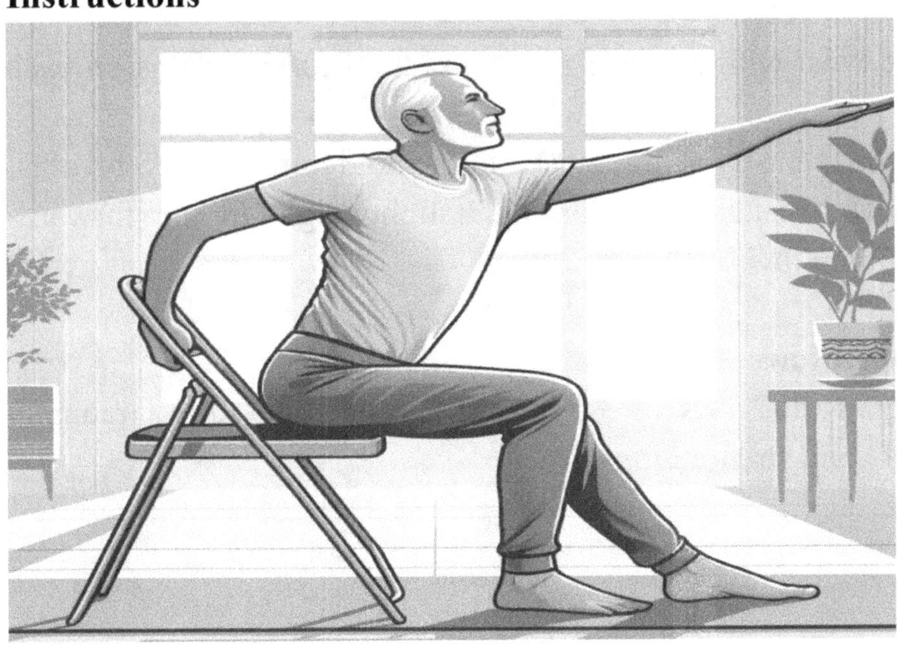

1. Starting Position: Sit upright in a sturdy, armless chair with your feet flat on the ground.

2. Execution: Place your right hand on the back of the chair. Inhale, and as you exhale, twist your torso to the right, reaching your left arm forward parallel to the floor. Turn your head to look over your left shoulder and also your right shoulder after some seconds if comfortable.

3. Hold and Breathe: Maintain this twisted position for a few deep breaths, focusing on stretching the spine with each exhale.

4. Release and Switch Sides: Return to the center on an inhale and repeat the twist on the opposite side.

Benefits

- Improves Spinal Flexibility: Regular practice increases flexibility and range of motion in the spine.
- Enhances Core Strength: Engages and strengthens the abdominal and back muscles.
- Reduces Back Pain: Helps alleviate tension and stiffness in the back and shoulders.
- Promotes Digestive Health: The twisting motion can stimulate digestion and help detoxify the organs.

Routine for Different Skill Levels
- Beginners: Perform the twist with a gentle reach and hold for 3 breaths on each side.
- Intermediate: Increase the intensity of the twist and the hold duration to 5 breaths.
- Advanced: Add a slight resistance by holding a lightweight in the forward-stretched hand, holding for up to 7 breaths.

Number of Sets and Repetitions
- General Guidance: Start with 2 sets of 3-5 repetitions on each side. Gradually increase as your flexibility and strength improve.

CHAIR SUPPORTED HALF MOON POSE

Introduction

The Chair Supported Half Moon Pose is an adaptation of the traditional Half Moon Pose, modified to provide stability and accessibility for seniors using a chair. This pose focuses on enhancing balance, flexibility, and strength in the side body, while also promoting mental focus.

Instructions

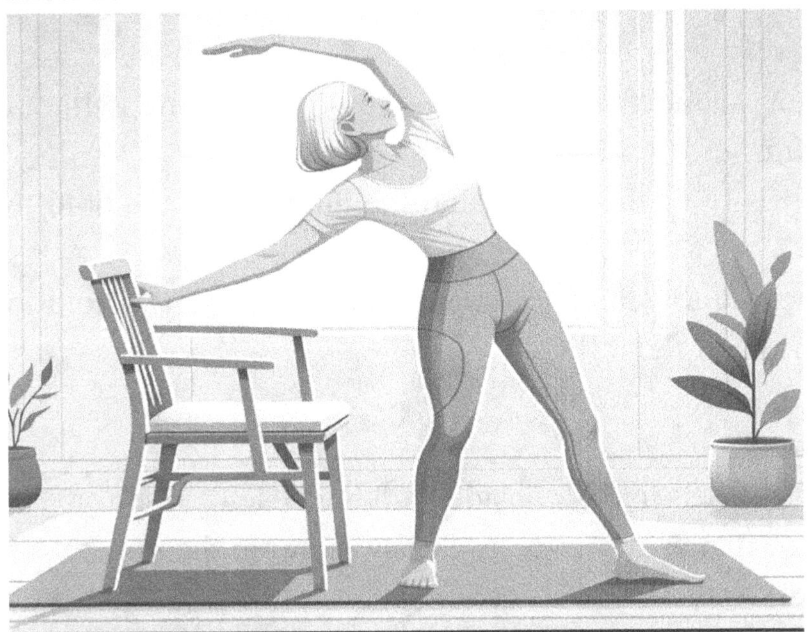

1. Starting Position: Stand next to a chair, placing it to your right side. Keep your feet flat and slightly apart for stability.

2. Execution: Place your right hand on the seat of the chair. Slowly lift your left arm overhead while simultaneously bending your torso to the right, over the chair. Extend your left arm fully to create a deep stretch along your left side. Your gaze can be directed forward or upward, depending on your neck comfort.

3. Hold and Breathe: Maintain this position for several deep breaths, focusing on stretching further with each exhale.

4. Release and Switch Sides: Gently come back to the starting position and repeat on the opposite side with the chair moved to your left.

Benefits

- Enhances Flexibility: Increases flexibility in the spine and lateral muscles of the torso.
- Improves Balance: Aids in developing balance and coordination, important for preventing falls.
- Strengthens Core Muscles: Engages the abdominal and oblique muscles, strengthening the core.
- Promotes Mental Focus: Requires concentration and body awareness, which can enhance overall mental clarity.

Routine for Different Skill Levels

- Beginners: Use the chair for support and focus on mild stretching without overexerting. Hold for 3-5 breaths.
- Intermediate: Increase the intensity of the stretch and the duration of the hold to 5-7 breaths.
- Advanced: Reduce the reliance on the chair for support and increase the hold to 8-10 breaths, challenging balance and flexibility.

Number of Sets and Repetitions

- General Guidance: Start with 2 sets on each side, holding each pose for 3-5 breaths. As your flexibility and balance improve, gradually increase the number of sets and the duration of each hold.

COOL DOWN EXERCISES

HAMSTRING STRETCH

Introduction
The Hamstring Stretch is an essential exercise for increasing flexibility in the back of the legs, particularly targeting the hamstring muscles. This stretch is crucial for seniors to maintain mobility, reduce the risk of injuries, and alleviate lower back pain.

Instructions

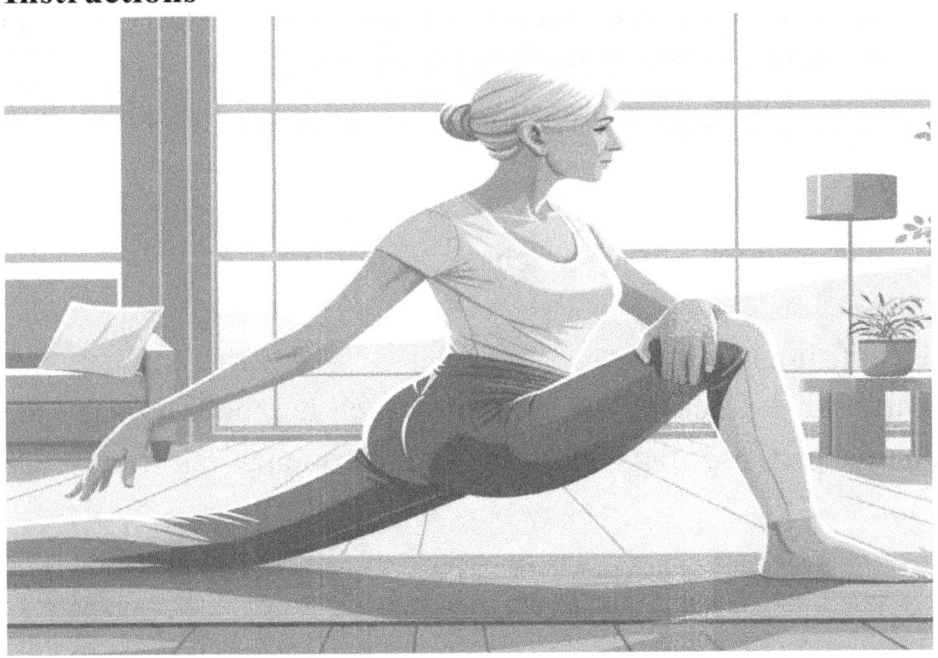

1. Starting Position: Sit on the floor or a mat with one leg extended straight ahead and the other leg bent, foot resting against the inner thigh of the extended leg.
2. Execution: Inhale and lengthen your spine. As you exhale, lean forward from your hips over the extended leg, reaching toward your toes with both hands. Keep your back straight and avoid rounding your shoulders.
3. Hold and Breathe: Hold this position for 15-30 seconds, breathing deeply to help relax into the stretch.

4. Release and Switch Sides: Gently come back up and switch legs to repeat the stretch on the other side.

Benefits
- Improves Flexibility: Enhances flexibility in the hamstrings, which can prevent injuries and improve functional movements like walking and bending.
- Reduces Lower Back Pain: Stretching the hamstrings relieves tension in the lower back, often a consequence of tight hamstrings.
- Enhances Circulation: Promotes blood flow to the lower body, which can aid in muscle recovery and health.
- Increases Mobility: Helps maintain a greater range of motion in the legs and hips.

Routine for Different Skill Levels
- Beginners: Focus on gentle stretches without forcing the torso towards the leg. Use a yoga strap or towel around the foot if unable to reach toes.
- Intermediate: Deepen the stretch by reaching further toward the foot and holding the position longer.
- Advanced: Attempt to lower the chest closer to the leg while maintaining a straight back, increasing the intensity of the stretch.

Number of Sets and Repetitions
- General Guidance: Start with 1-2 sets of the stretch on each leg, holding each for 15-30 seconds. Gradually increase the duration and frequency as flexibility improves.

COBRA POSE

Introduction

The Cobra Pose, or Bhujangasana, is a gentle backbend that strengthens the spine, opens the chest, shoulders, and abdomen, and is often incorporated into yoga routines for its health benefits. This exercise is particularly suitable for seniors as it can help improve flexibility and posture.

Instructions

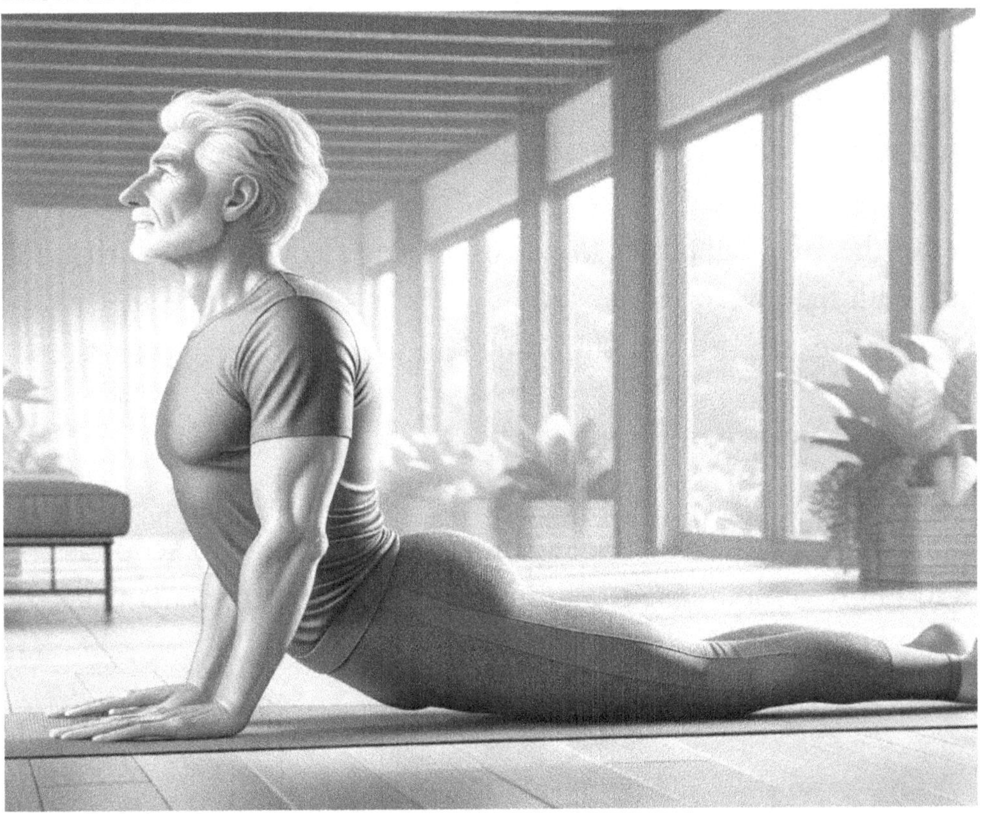

1. Starting Position: Lie face down on a yoga mat with your legs extended behind you, tops of the feet pressing down into the mat.
2. Execution: Place your hands under your shoulders with your elbows close to your body. Gradually lift your chest off the mat by straightening your arms, keeping your hips and legs pressed down. Tilt your head slightly upwards, maintaining a gentle gaze forward.
3. Hold and Breathe: Hold the pose for 15-30 seconds, taking slow and deep breaths to help open up your chest and relax into the stretch.
4. Release: Slowly lower your chest back to the mat and relax.

Benefits
- Strengthens the Spine: Regular practice helps strengthen the muscles of the back and spine.
- Increases Flexibility: Improves flexibility in the back and shoulders, aiding in the relief of tension and pain.
- Stimulates Abdominal Organs: The pose encourages abdominal stretching, which can help stimulate abdominal organs and improve digestion.
- Elevates Mood: Helps in reducing stress and fatigue, promoting a sense of well-being.

Routine for Different Skill Levels
- Beginners: Focus on lifting only to a comfortable height, maintaining a slight bend in the elbows.
- Intermediate: Increase the lift, extending the arms more fully while ensuring the hips remain in contact with the mat.
- Advanced: Hold the pose for longer durations and experiment with deeper backbends, if comfortable.

Number of Sets and Repetitions
- General Guidance: Start with 2-3 repetitions, holding each for 15-30 seconds. As flexibility and strength improve, increase the duration and number of repetitions.

SEATED GENTLE NECK STRETCHES

Introduction
Seated Gentle Neck Stretches are crucial for seniors looking to relieve tension and improve flexibility in the neck area. This exercise is designed to be gentle and safe, making it ideal for those with limited mobility or who spend long periods sitting.

Instructions

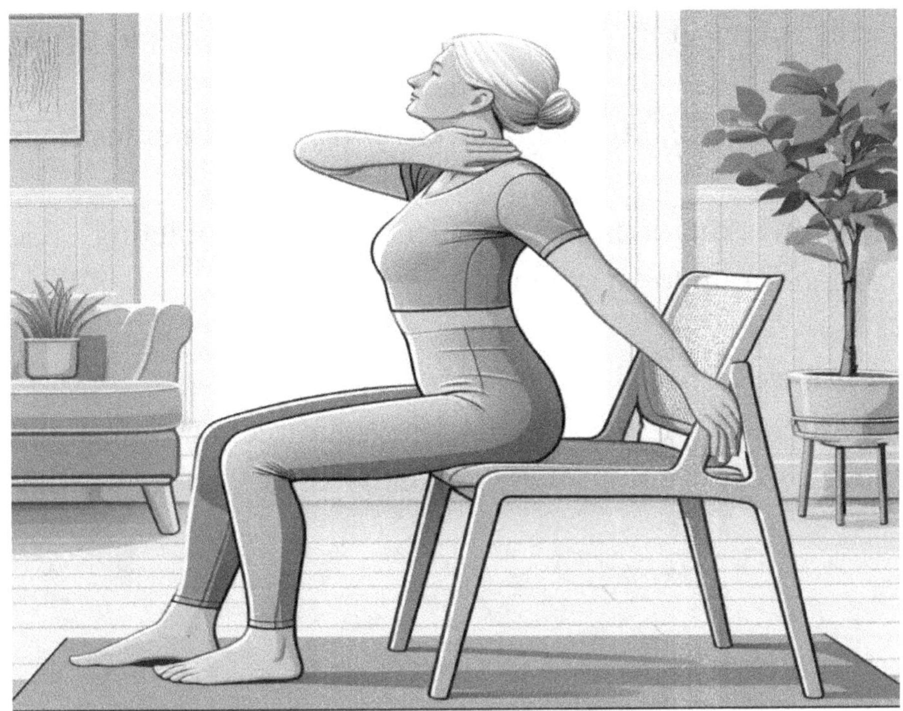

1. Starting Position: Sit upright in a chair without arms, feet flat on the floor.
2. Execution: Gently tilt your head to one side, bringing your ear towards your shoulder. Hold this position for a few seconds, feeling a stretch on the opposite side of your neck.
3. Switch Sides: Slowly return your head to the center and repeat the stretch on the other side.
4. Forward and Backward: Gently nod your head forward, trying to touch your chin to your chest, and then tilt your head backward, looking up at the ceiling.

Benefits

- Improves Flexibility: Increases flexibility in the neck, which can reduce pain and stiffness.
- Relieves Tension: Helps alleviate tension and stress accumulated in the neck muscles.
- Enhances Circulation: Promotes better blood circulation to the neck area.
- Increases Range of Motion: Regular stretching can help maintain a healthy range of motion in the cervical spine.

Routine for Different Skill Levels

- Beginners: Perform each stretch for about 5 seconds, focusing on gentle movements without straining.
- Intermediate: Hold each stretch for 10 seconds, ensuring smooth transitions between movements.
- Advanced: Incorporate gentle rotations of the neck after completing side stretches, holding each position for up to 15 seconds.

Number of Sets and Repetitions
- General Guidance: Start with 2 sets of 3 repetitions for each direction (left, right, forward, backward). As your flexibility improves, gradually increase the duration and number of sets.

WORKOUT PLANNER(28 DAYS YOGA CHALLENGE)

Week 1: The Foundation work

Day 1:
- Morning Routine (5-7 minutes):
  - Warm-Up: Seated Marching Exercise - 1 minute (Improves circulation and warms up the legs)
  - Main Exercise: Chair Warrior I - 2 minutes (Increases flexibility and strength in the legs and core)
  - Cool Down: Hamstring Stretch - 2 minutes (Reduces stiffness in the back of the legs)

- Evening Routine (5-7 minutes):
  - Warm-Up: Ankle Flex and Point Exercise - 1 minute (Enhances ankle mobility and circulation)
  - Main Exercise: Seated Forward Bend - 3 minutes (Promotes spinal flexibility and calms the nervous system)
  - Cool Down: Seated Gentle Neck Stretches - 1 minute (Relieves neck tension)

Day 2:
- Morning Routine (5-7 minutes):
  - Warm-Up: Wrist and Finger Stretch Exercise - 1 minute (Increases flexibility in hands and wrists)
  - Main Exercise: Chair Extended Side Angle - 3 minutes (Improves side body stretching, enhances posture)

- Cool Down: Shoulder Circle Exercise - 1 minute (Loosens shoulder joints)

- Evening Routine (5-7 minutes):
  - Warm-Up: Shoulder Blade Squeeze - 1 minute (Strengthens back muscles, improves posture)
  - Main Exercise: Seated Side Bends - 3 minutes (Enhances core stability and lateral flexibility)
  - Cool Down: Cobra Pose - 1 minute (Strengthens the spine, soothes sciatica)

Day 3:

- Morning Routine (5-7 minutes):
  - Warm-Up: Seated Cat-Cow Stretch - 1 minute (Increases spine flexibility)
  - Main Exercise: Chair Pigeon Pose - 3 minutes (Opens the hips, improves lower body flexibility)
  - Cool Down: Seated Chest Opener - 1 minute (Enhances breathing, opens up chest and shoulders)

- Evening Routine (5-7 minutes):
  - Warm-Up: Seated Hip Marching - 1 minute (Activates the hip joints)
  - Main Exercise: Chair Plank Pose - 3 minutes (Builds core strength, enhances stability)
  - Cool Down: Seated Gentle Neck Stretches - 1 minute

Day 4:

- Morning Routine (5-7 minutes):
  - Warm-Up: Side Neck Stretch Exercise - 1 minute (Relieves tension and improves neck flexibility)
  - Main Exercise: Chair Pelvic Tilts - 3 minutes (Strengthens the core, improves lower back health)
  - Cool Down: Seated Knee to Chest - 1 minute (Relaxes the lower back, enhances hip flexibility)

- Evening Routine (5-7 minutes):

- Warm-Up: Shoulder Circle Exercise - 1 minute (Improves shoulder mobility)
- Main Exercise: Seated Spinal Twist with Arm Reach - 3 minutes (Enhances spinal mobility, aids in digestion)
- Cool Down: Cobra Pose - 1 minute (Strengthens the lower back, opens the chest)

Day 5:
- Morning Routine (5-7 minutes):
- Warm-Up: Ankle Rotations - 1 minute (Increases ankle mobility, reduces stiffness)
- Main Exercise: Chair Boat Pose - 3 minutes (Builds core strength, enhances balance)
- Cool Down: Hamstring Stretch - 1 minute (Improves flexibility in the hamstrings, eases tension in the back)

- Evening Routine (5-7 minutes):
- Warm-Up: Seated Chest Opener - 1 minute (Expands the chest, improves breathing capacity)
- Main Exercise: Chair Supported Half Moon Pose - 3 minutes (Promotes balance and stability, strengthens the core)
- Cool Down: Seated Gentle Neck Stretches - 1 minute (Relieves neck and shoulder tension)

Day 6:
- Morning Routine (5-7 minutes):
- Warm-Up: Wrist and Finger Stretch Exercise - 1 minute (Prepares hands and wrists for activity)
- Main Exercise: Seated Leg Extensions - 3 minutes (Strengthens thighs, enhances leg flexibility)
- Cool Down: Seated Forward Bend - 1 minute (Calms the mind, stretches the spine)

- Evening Routine (5-7 minutes):
  - Warm-Up: Seated Hip Marching - 1 minute (Activates the hip flexors)
  - Main Exercise: Chair Assisted Triangle Pose - 3 minutes (Improves side-body stretch, enhances posture)
  - Cool Down: Cobra Pose - 1 minute

Day 7:

- Morning Routine (5-7 minutes):
  - Warm-Up: Ankle Flex and Point Exercise - 1 minute (Improves circulation and ankle mobility)
  - Main Exercise: Overhead Arm Clasp - 3 minutes (Stretches the shoulders and improves upper body mobility)
  - Cool Down: Seated Gentle Neck Stretches - 1 minute

- Evening Routine (5-7 minutes):
  - Warm-Up: Shoulder Blade Squeeze - 1 minute (Strengthens the upper back, corrects posture)
  - Main Exercise: Seated Cat-Cow Stretch - 3 minutes (Increases spinal flexibility, relieves tension in the torso)
  - Cool Down: Seated Knee to Chest - 1 minute

Week 2: The Building Block

Each session still targets a warm-up, a main exercise, and a cool-down, focusing on building upon the foundational work from Week 1 and introducing new exercises to keep the routine engaging and effective.

Day 8:

- Morning Routine (5-7 minutes):
  - Warm-Up: Seated Marching Exercise - 1 minute (Activates leg muscles, stimulates circulation)

- Main Exercise: Chair Warrior I - 3 minutes (Builds strength and flexibility in legs and core)
   - Cool Down: Seated Forward Bend - 1 minute (Stretches the back, promotes relaxation)

- Evening Routine (5-7 minutes):
   - Warm-Up: Ankle Flex and Point Exercise - 1 minute (Enhances ankle flexibility, promotes circulation)
   - Main Exercise: Chair Pigeon Pose - 3 minutes (Improves hip flexibility, reduces lower back pain)
   - Cool Down: Hamstring Stretch - 1 minute (Eases tension in the back of the legs)

Day 9:

- Morning Routine (5-7 minutes):
   - Warm-Up: Wrist and Finger Stretch Exercise - 1 minute (Increases hand and wrist mobility)
   - Main Exercise: Chair Extended Side Angle - 3 minutes (Enhances lateral body stretch, improves posture)
   - Cool Down: Shoulder Circle Exercise - 1 minute (Improves shoulder flexibility and reduces stiffness)

- Evening Routine (5-7 minutes):
   - Warm-Up: Shoulder Blade Squeeze - 1 minute (Improves posture, strengthens back muscles)
   - Main Exercise: Seated Side Bends - 3 minutes (Builds core strength, enhances flexibility)
   - Cool Down: Cobra Pose - 1 minute (Strengthens the spine, improves flexibility)

Day 10:

- Morning Routine (5-7 minutes):
   - Warm-Up: Seated Cat-Cow Stretch - 1 minute (Enhances spine mobility)
   - Main Exercise: Chair Boat Pose - 3 minutes (Strengthens the core, improves balance)

- Cool Down: Seated Chest Opener - 1 minute (Opens up the chest, enhances lung capacity)

- Evening Routine (5-7 minutes):
  - Warm-Up: Seated Hip Marching - 1 minute (Activates hips and core)
  - Main Exercise: Chair Plank Pose - 3 minutes (Builds core stability, strengthens arms and shoulders)
  - Cool Down: Seated Gentle Neck Stretches - 1 minute (Relieves neck tension)

Day 11:
- Morning Routine (5-7 minutes):
  - Warm-Up: Ankle Rotations - 1 minute (Improves ankle mobility)
  - Main Exercise: Seated Spinal Twist with Arm Reach - 3 minutes (Enhances spinal mobility, aids digestion)
  - Cool Down: Shoulder Circle Exercise - 1 minute (Loosens and relaxes shoulder joints)

- Evening Routine (5-7 minutes):
  - Warm-Up: Side Neck Stretch Exercise - 1 minute (Relieves neck tension)
  - Main Exercise: Chair Assisted Triangle Pose - 3 minutes (Improves balance, stretches side body)
  - Cool Down: Cobra Pose - 1 minute (Opens the chest, strengthens the lower back)

Day 12:
- Morning Routine (5-7 minutes):
  - Warm-Up: Seated Marching Exercise - 1 minute
  - Main Exercise: Overhead Arm Clasp - 3 minutes (Improves shoulder flexibility, opens up chest)
  - Cool Down: Hamstring Stretch - 1 minute (Relaxes hamstrings, improves leg flexibility)

- Evening Routine (5-7 minutes):

- Warm-Up: Wrist and Finger Stretch Exercise - 1 minute
- Main Exercise: Seated Leg Extensions - 3 minutes (Strengthens thighs, enhances knee mobility)
- Cool Down: Seated Gentle Neck Stretches - 1 minute

Day 13:
- Morning Routine (5-7 minutes):
  - Warm-Up: Shoulder Circle Exercise - 1 minute
  - Main Exercise: Seated Knee to Chest - 3 minutes (Enhances hip flexibility, relieves lower back tension)
  - Cool Down: Seated Forward Bend - 1 minute

- Evening Routine (5-7 minutes):
  - Warm-Up: Ankle Flex and Point Exercise

 - 1 minute
  - Main Exercise: Chair Supported Half Moon Pose - 3 minutes (Enhances balance, strengthens obliques)
  - Cool Down: Cobra Pose - 1 minute

Day 14:
- Morning Routine (5-7 minutes):
  - Warm-Up: Ankle Rotations - 1 minute
  - Main Exercise: Chair Pelvic Tilts - 3 minutes (Strengthens core, improves lower back flexibility)
  - Cool Down: Seated Chest Opener - 1 minute

- Evening Routine (5-7 minutes):
  - Warm-Up: Shoulder Blade Squeeze - 1 minute
  - Main Exercise: Seated Cat-Cow Stretch - 3 minutes (Increases spinal flexibility, relaxes torso)
  - Cool Down: Seated Gentle Neck Stretches - 1 minute

This plan for Days 8 to 14 contains different exercises each day, ensuring a balanced routine that targets various aspects of physical health, such as flexibility, strength, and balance, with careful attention to warm-ups and cool-downs to prepare for and recover from each session.

Week 3: Slow Advancement

For the third week of your 28-Day Chair Yoga Challenge, we'll continue to vary the exercises each day, focusing on more integration of the exercises practiced in previous weeks and emphasizing on deepening the stretches and strengthening the core muscles further.

In this level you can advance the pose and even increase the duration of the exercise.

Day 15:

- Morning Routine (5-7 minutes):
  - Warm-Up: Seated Marching Exercise - 1 minute (Stimulates circulation and warms up the legs)
  - Main Exercise: Chair Warrior I - 3 minutes (Builds lower body strength and improves balance)
  - Cool Down: Seated Forward Bend - 1 minute (Calms the mind, stretches the spine)

- Evening Routine (5-7 minutes):
  - Warm-Up: Ankle Flex and Point Exercise - 1 minute (Enhances ankle flexibility, promotes circulation)
  - Main Exercise: Chair Pigeon Pose - 3 minutes (Opens hips, improves lower body flexibility)
  - Cool Down: Hamstring Stretch - 1 minute (Eases stiffness in hamstrings)

Day 16:

- Morning Routine (5-7 minutes):

- Warm-Up: Wrist and Finger Stretch Exercise - 1 minute (Increases mobility in hands and wrists)
  - Main Exercise: Chair Extended Side Angle - 3 minutes (Enhances lateral body stretch, improves posture)
  - Cool Down: Shoulder Circle Exercise - 1 minute (Improves shoulder flexibility and reduces stiffness)

- Evening Routine (5-7 minutes):
  - Warm-Up: Shoulder Blade Squeeze - 1 minute (Strengthens back muscles, improves posture)
  - Main Exercise: Seated Side Bends - 3 minutes (Enhances core strength, increases lateral flexibility)
  - Cool Down: Cobra Pose - 1 minute (Strengthens the lower back, improves spinal flexibility)

Day 17:
- Morning Routine (5-7 minutes):
  - Warm-Up: Seated Cat-Cow Stretch - 1 minute (Enhances spinal mobility)
  - Main Exercise: Chair Boat Pose - 3 minutes (Strengthens core muscles, improves balance)
  - Cool Down: Seated Chest Opener - 1 minute (Opens the chest, enhances lung capacity)

- Evening Routine (5-7 minutes):
  - Warm-Up: Seated Hip Marching - 1 minute (Activates hips and core)
  - Main Exercise: Chair Plank Pose - 3 minutes (Strengthens arms and core, increases overall stability)
  - Cool Down: Seated Gentle Neck Stretches - 1 minute (Relieves tension in the neck)

Day 18:
- Morning Routine (5-7 minutes):
  - Warm-Up: Ankle Rotations - 1 minute (Improves ankle mobility)

- Main Exercise: Seated Spinal Twist with Arm Reach - 3 minutes (Enhances spinal flexibility, aids digestion)
  - Cool Down: Shoulder Circle Exercise - 1 minute (Relaxes shoulder joints)

- Evening Routine (5-7 minutes):
  - Warm-Up: Side Neck Stretch Exercise - 1 minute (Relieves neck tension)
  - Main Exercise: Chair Assisted Triangle Pose - 3 minutes (Improves balance, stretches the torso)
  - Cool Down: Cobra Pose - 1 minute (Opens the chest, strengthens the spine)

Day 19:
- Morning Routine (5-7 minutes):
  - Warm-Up: Seated Marching Exercise - 1 minute
  - Main Exercise: Overhead Arm Clasp - 3 minutes (Improves shoulder flexibility, opens the upper back)
  - Cool Down: Hamstring Stretch - 1 minute (Improves flexibility in the hamstrings)

- Evening Routine (5-7 minutes):
  - Warm-Up: Wrist and Finger Stretch Exercise - 1 minute
  - Main Exercise: Seated Leg Extensions - 3 minutes (Strengthens thigh muscles, enhances leg flexibility)
  - Cool Down: Seated Gentle Neck Stretches - 1 minute (Eases neck tension)

Day 20:
- Morning Routine (5-7 minutes):
  - Warm-Up: Shoulder Circle Exercise - 1 minute
  - Main Exercise: Seated Knee to Chest - 3 minutes (Enhances hip flexibility, relieves lower back tension)
  - Cool Down: Seated Forward Bend - 1 minute (Stretches the back, promotes relaxation)

- Evening Routine (5-7 minutes):

- Warm-Up: Ankle Flex and Point Exercise - 1 minute
  - Main Exercise: Chair Supported Half Moon Pose - 3 minutes (Enhances balance, strengthens the core and side body)
  - Cool Down: Cobra Pose - 1 minute

Day 21:

- Morning Routine (5-7 minutes):
  - Warm-Up: Ankle Rotations - 1 minute
  - Main Exercise: Chair Pelvic Tilts - 3 minutes (Strengthens core, improves posture)
  - Cool Down: Seated Chest Opener - 1 minute (Expands the chest, improves breathing)

- Evening Routine (5-7 minutes):
  - Warm-Up: Shoulder Blade Squeeze - 1 minute
  - Main Exercise: Seated Cat-Cow Stretch - 3 minutes (Increases spine flexibility, calms the mind)
  - Cool Down: Seated Gentle Neck Stretches - 1 minute

This weekly plan continues to develop the core principles of chair yoga—flexibility, balance, strength, and relaxation—while ensuring variety and progression to keep the practice engaging and effective.

Week 4: Advanced Level

For the final week of your 28-Day Chair Yoga Challenge, we'll continue to diversify the exercises while emphasizing mastering the movements and deepening the stretches. This week will consolidate all that has been learned, allowing participants to truly benefit from increased flexibility, strength, and relaxation.

Day 22:

- Morning Routine (5-7 minutes):
  - Warm-Up: Seated Marching Exercise - 1 minute (Activates leg muscles and stimulates circulation)
  - Main Exercise: Chair Warrior I - 3 minutes (Strengthens legs and improves balance)
  - Cool Down: Seated Forward Bend - 1 minute (Stretches the spine, promotes relaxation)

- Evening Routine (5-7 minutes):
  - Warm-Up: Ankle Flex and Point Exercise - 1 minute (Enhances ankle flexibility)
  - Main Exercise: Chair Pigeon Pose - 3 minutes (Opens the hips, improves flexibility)
  - Cool Down: Hamstring Stretch - 1 minute (Eases stiffness in the back of legs)

Day 23:

- Morning Routine (5-7 minutes):
  - Warm-Up: Wrist and Finger Stretch Exercise - 1 minute (Increases mobility in hands and wrists)
  - Main Exercise: Chair Extended Side Angle - 3 minutes (Improves lateral body stretch and posture)
  - Cool Down: Shoulder Circle Exercise - 1 minute (Lowers shoulder tension)

- Evening Routine (5-7 minutes):
  - Warm-Up: Shoulder Blade Squeeze - 1 minute (Improves upper back posture)
  - Main Exercise: Seated Side Bends - 3 minutes (Strengthens obliques and core)
  - Cool Down: Cobra Pose - 1 minute (Strengthens the spine)

Day 24:

- Morning Routine (5-7 minutes):
  - Warm-Up: Seated Cat-Cow Stretch - 1 minute (Enhances spinal flexibility)

- Main Exercise: Chair Boat Pose - 3 minutes (Strengthens the core, improves balance)
  - Cool Down: Seated Chest Opener - 1 minute (Enhances lung capacity, opens chest)

- Evening Routine (5-7 minutes):
  - Warm-Up: Seated Hip Marching - 1 minute (Activates hip joints)
  - Main Exercise: Chair Plank Pose - 3 minutes (Increases core and arm strength)
  - Cool Down: Seated Gentle Neck Stretches - 1 minute (Relieves neck strain)

Day 25:
- Morning Routine (5-7 minutes):
  - Warm-Up: Ankle Rotations - 1 minute (Increases ankle mobility)
  - Main Exercise: Seated Spinal Twist with Arm Reach - 3 minutes (Enhances spinal rotation, aids digestion)
  - Cool Down: Shoulder Circle Exercise - 1 minute (Relaxes shoulders)

- Evening Routine (5-7 minutes):
  - Warm-Up: Side Neck Stretch Exercise - 1 minute (Relieves neck tension)
  - Main Exercise: Chair Assisted Triangle Pose - 3 minutes (Improves balance, stretches torso)
  - Cool Down: Cobra Pose - 1 minute (Strengthens lower back)

Day 26:
- Morning Routine (5-7 minutes):
  - Warm-Up: Seated Marching Exercise - 1 minute
  - Main Exercise: Overhead Arm Clasp - 3 minutes (Improves shoulder flexibility, opens upper back)
  - Cool Down: Hamstring Stretch - 1 minute (Improves leg flexibility)

- Evening Routine (5-7 minutes):
  - Warm-Up: Wrist and Finger Stretch Exercise - 1 minute

- Main Exercise: Seated Leg Extensions - 3 minutes (Strengthens thighs, improves knee mobility)
  - Cool Down: Seated Gentle Neck Stretches - 1 minute

Day 27:
- Morning Routine (5-7 minutes):
  - Warm-Up: Shoulder Circle Exercise - 1 minute
  - Main Exercise: Seated Knee to Chest - 3 minutes (Enhances hip flexibility, relieves lower back tension)
  - Cool Down: Seated Forward Bend - 1 minute (Calms the mind, stretches the back)

- Evening Routine (5-7 minutes):
  - Warm-Up: Ankle Flex and Point Exercise - 1 minute
  - Main Exercise: Chair Supported Half Moon Pose - 3 minutes (Improves balance and core strength)
  - Cool Down: Cobra Pose -
  1 minute

Day 28:
- Morning Routine (5-7 minutes):
  - Warm-Up: Ankle Rotations - 1 minute
  - Main Exercise: Chair Pelvic Tilts - 3 minutes (Strengthens core, improves lower back flexibility)
  - Cool Down: Seated Chest Opener - 1 minute (Expands chest, improves breathing)

- Evening Routine (5-7 minutes):
  - Warm-Up: Shoulder Blade Squeeze - 1 minute
  - Main Exercise: Seated Cat-Cow Stretch - 3 minutes (Increases spine flexibility, soothes the torso)
  - Cool Down: Seated Gentle Neck Stretches - 1 minute

This final week's plan builds on the consistency and progress made throughout the challenge, refining technique and deepening stretches to maximize the benefits of chair yoga. The last day of the challenge is designed to encapsulate all the elements of flexibility, balance, strength, and relaxation, ensuring a comprehensive and rewarding yoga practice.

Additional Customizable Workout Planner

After completing the 28-Days challenge you have the better ideas of what your body can take and not take. With your experience so far you now know exercises that are suitable for you and the one's you least prefer. With the knowledge you can set up your own workout plan that suit you best and help the best results.

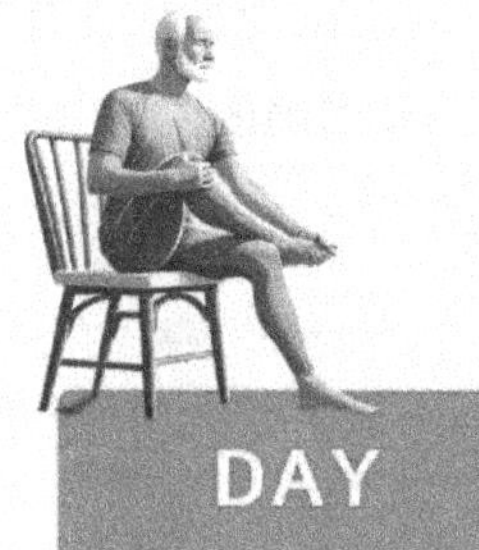

CHAIR YOGA WORKOUT PLANNER

DAY	EXERCISE	DURATION
Monday		
Tuesday		
Wednesday		
Thursday		
Friday		
Saturday		
Sunday		

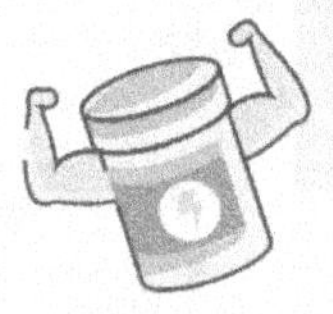

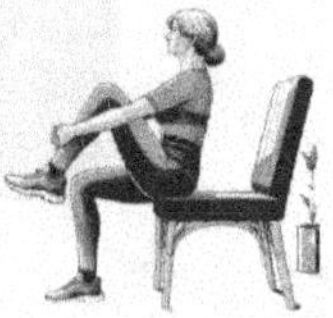

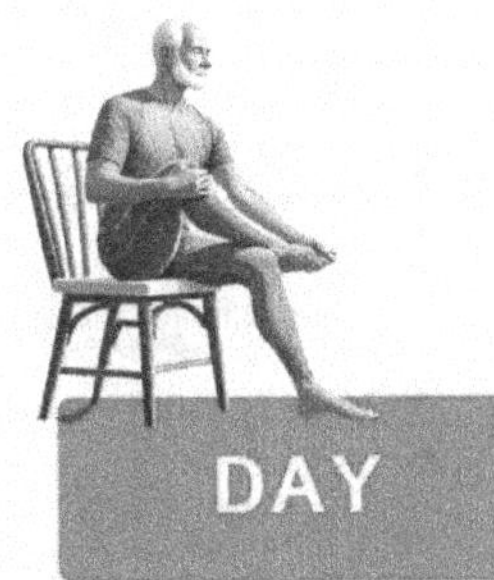

DAY	EXERCISE	DURATION
Monday		
Tuesday		
Wednesday		
Thursday		
Friday		
Saturday		
Sunday		

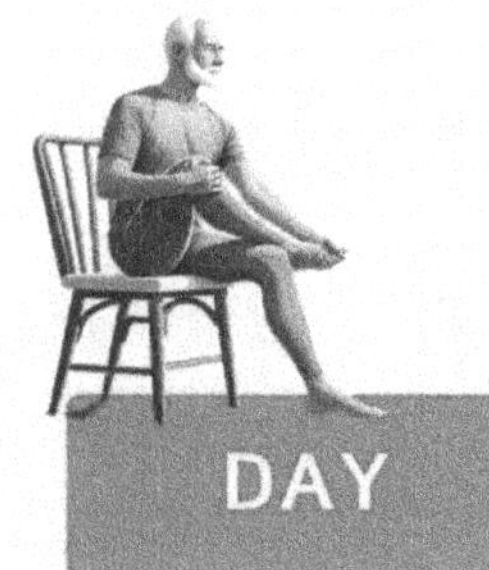

DAY	EXERCISE	DURATION
Monday		
Tuesday		
Wednesday		
Thursday		
Friday		
Saturday		
Sunday		

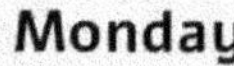
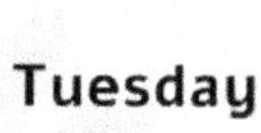
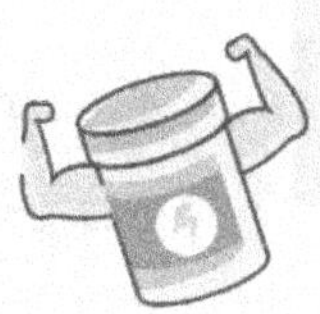
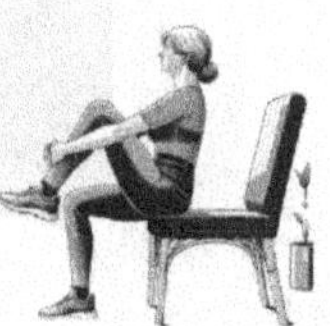

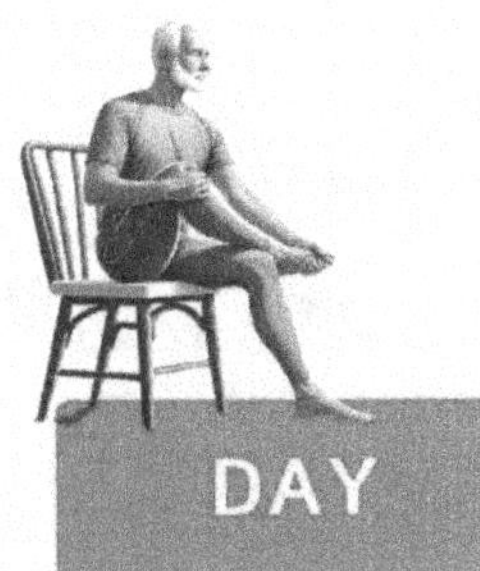

CHAIR YOGA WORKOUT PLANNER

DAY	EXERCISE	DURATION
Monday		
Tuesday		
Wednesday		
Thursday		
Friday		
Saturday		
Sunday		

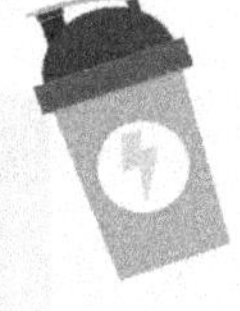

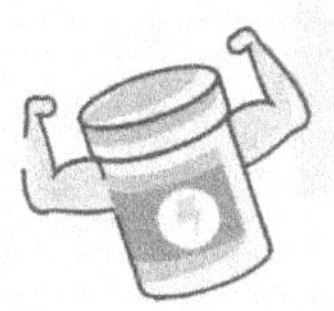

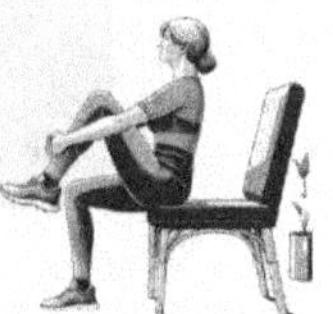

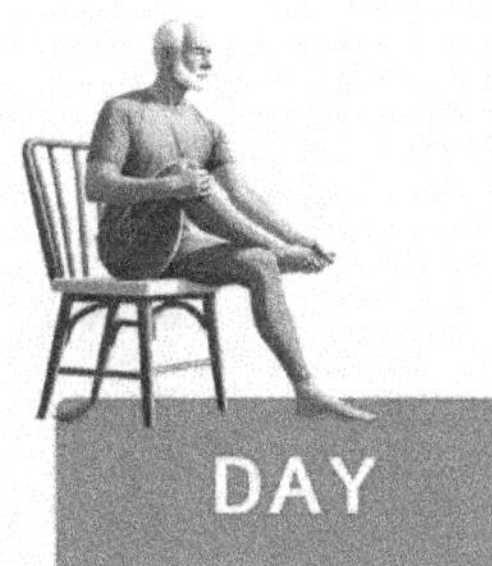

CHAIR YOGA WORKOUT PLANNER

DAY	EXERCISE	DURATION
Monday		
Tuesday		
Wednesday		
Thursday		
Friday		
Saturday		
Sunday		

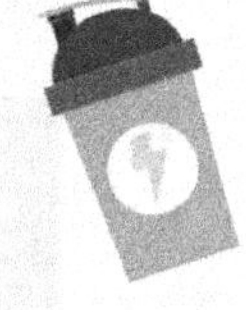

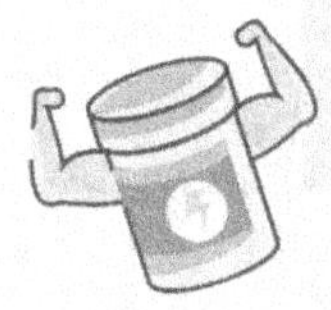

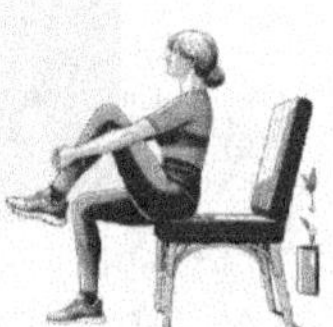

CHAIR YOGA WORKOUT PLANNER

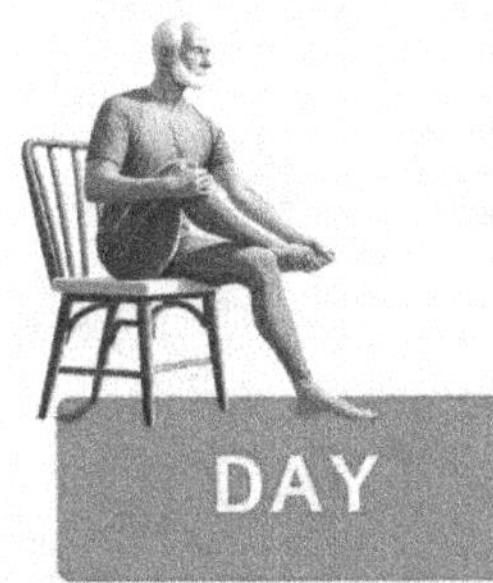

DAY	EXERCISE	DURATION
Monday		
Tuesday		
Wednesday		
Thursday		
Friday		
Saturday		
Sunday		

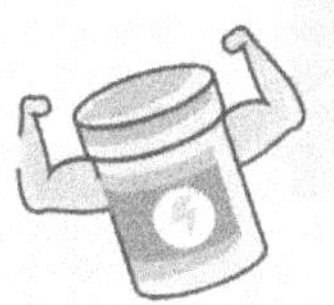

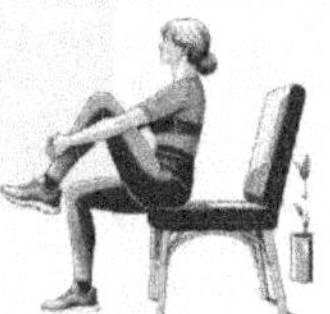

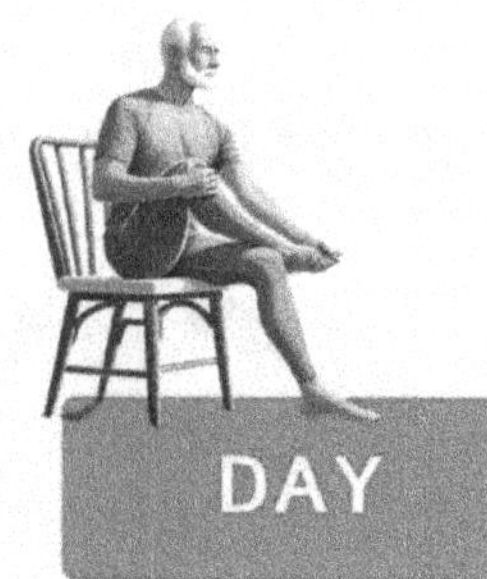

CHAIR YOGA WORKOUT PLANNER

DAY	EXERCISE	DURATION
Monday		
Tuesday		
Wednesday		
Thursday		
Friday		
Saturday		
Sunday		

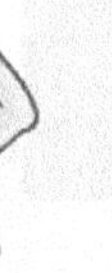

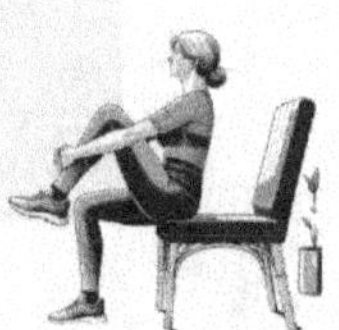

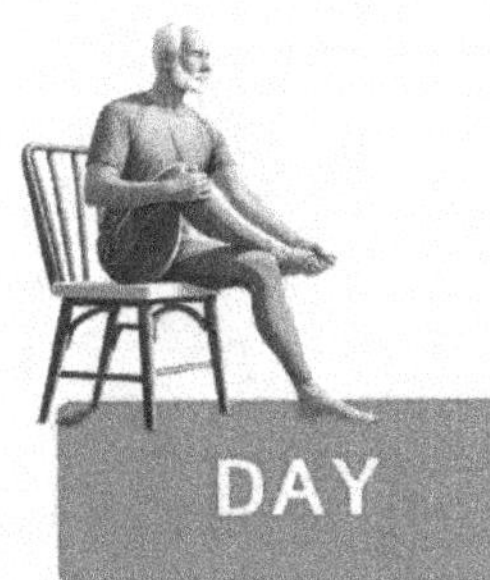

CHAIR YOGA WORKOUT PLANNER

DAY	EXERCISE	DURATION
Monday		
Tuesday		
Wednesday		
Thursday		
Friday		
Saturday		
Sunday		

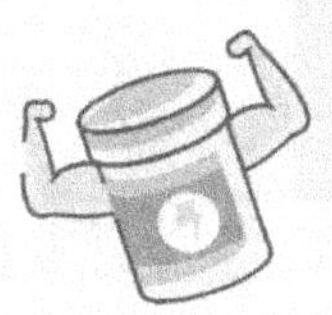

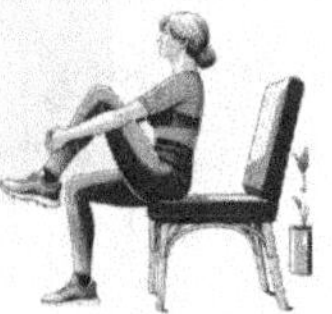

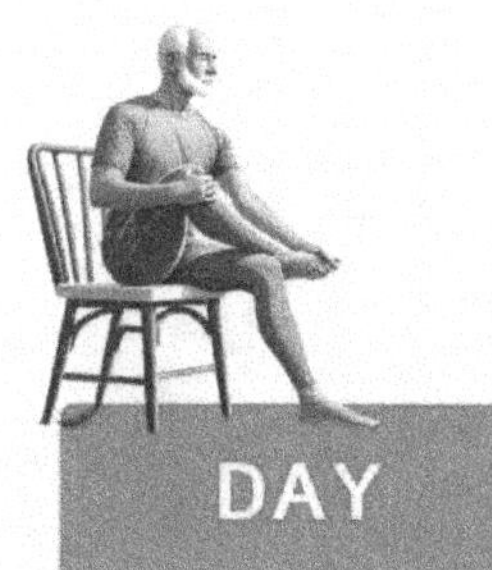

CHAIR YOGA WORKOUT PLANNER

DAY	EXERCISE	DURATION
Monday		
Tuesday		
Wednesday		
Thursday		
Friday		
Saturday		
Sunday		

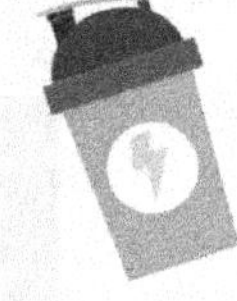

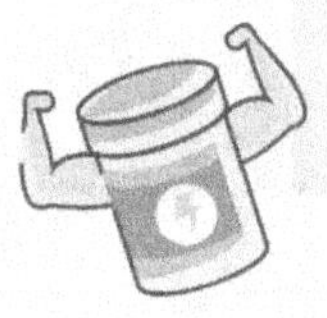

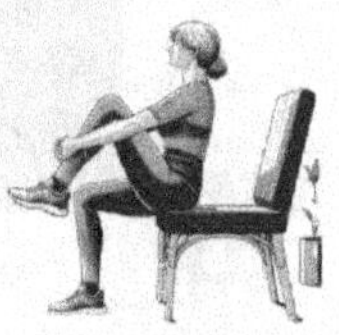

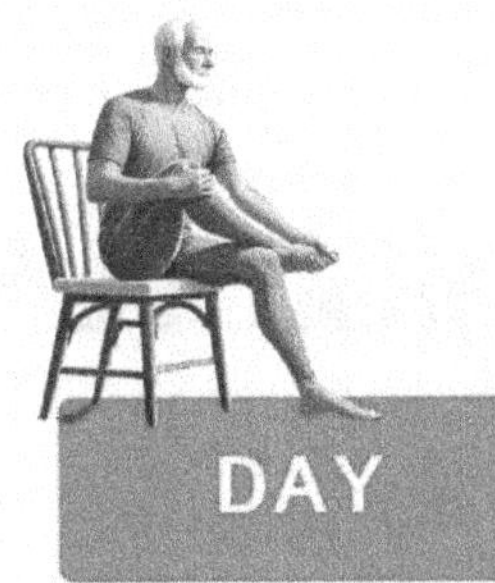

CHAIR YOGA WORKOUT PLANNER

DAY	EXERCISE	DURATION
Monday		
Tuesday		
Wednesday		
Thursday		
Friday		
Saturday		
Sunday		

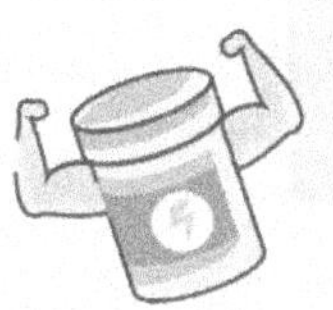

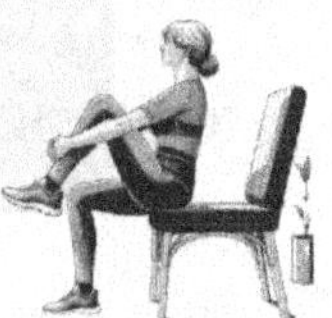

SHOPPING LIST AND PROPER MEAL PLAN

Shopping List

This list will help ensure you have everything needed to prepare these nutritious meals, supporting a healthy lifestyle alongside chair yoga activities.

Dairy & Eggs:
- Greek yogurt
- Milk (or almond milk)
- Eggs
- Feta cheese
- Cheddar cheese

Proteins:
- Cooked chicken breast
- Salmon fillets
- Lean beef strips
- Turkey breast cubes
- Canned tuna (in water)
- Mixed beans (canned or dry)

Grains:
- Rolled oats
- Quinoa
- Whole grain bread
- Brown rice

Vegetables:
- Mixed berries (fresh or frozen)
- Fresh spinach

- Avocado
- Celery
- Broccoli
- Onion
- Bell peppers (various colors)
- Carrots
- Sweet potatoes
- Mixed vegetables (for stir-fry)
- Tomatoes
- Garlic
- Zucchini
- Brussels sprouts
- Lettuce
- Cucumber

Fruits:
- Lemons
- Apples
- Fresh fruit for parfaits (e.g., berries, banana)

Nuts & Seeds:
- Mixed nuts (e.g., almonds, walnuts)

Herbs & Spices:
- Cinnamon
- Fresh dill
- Herbs (rosemary, thyme, cilantro)
- Chili spices

Oils & Condiments:
- Olive oil
- Vegetable broth
- Sesame oil
- Soy sauce
- Honey or maple syrup

- Greek yogurt (as a dressing/sauce base)
- Mustard
- Lime (for dressing)

Miscellaneous:
- Salt and pepper

This list includes a wide range of ingredients to provide varied and balanced nutrition, catering specifically to the needs of seniors engaged in physical activities like chair yoga. Adjust quantities based on your meal planning and number of servings required.

Foods to Avoid for Seniors in a Chair Yoga Program

For seniors participating in a chair yoga program, maintaining a diet that supports flexibility, joint health, and overall wellness is crucial. It's equally important to avoid certain foods that may hinder their health or exacerbate existing conditions. Here are some types of foods that seniors should generally avoid or consume minimally:

1. High-Sodium Foods:
   - Avoid processed meats, canned soups, and ready meals that typically contain high levels of sodium, which can lead to high blood pressure and fluid retention, affecting heart health and joint swelling.

2. Sugary Foods and Beverages:
   - Limit or avoid sodas, sugary snacks, and desserts like cakes and candies. Excessive sugar can lead to weight gain, exacerbate diabetes, and result in energy crashes that might affect their yoga practice.

3. Excessive Caffeine:

- While a moderate amount of coffee or tea can be beneficial, too much caffeine can interfere with sleep patterns and bone health. Seniors should limit coffee, strong tea, and energy drinks.

4. Refined Carbohydrates:
- Foods like white bread, pastries, and other products made from refined flour can lead to increased blood sugar levels and are not beneficial for energy stability.

5. Fried and High-Fat Foods:
- Reduce intake of deep-fried foods and dishes high in saturated fats such as fatty cuts of meat, butter, and high-fat dairy. These can contribute to cholesterol levels and cardiovascular issues.

6. Alcohol:
- Limit alcohol consumption as it can interfere with sleep quality and medication effectiveness. Alcohol can also contribute to dehydration and bone density loss.

7. Raw Undercooked Foods:
- Seniors should be cautious with raw or undercooked meats, seafood, and eggs due to a higher risk of foodborne illnesses which can be more severe in older adults.

8. Artificial Sweeteners and Additives:
- Minimize foods with artificial sweeteners and additives, as they can have laxative effects and may affect digestive health.

By avoiding these types of foods, seniors can better manage their health conditions and maintain the energy and mobility needed to actively participate in chair yoga and other physical activities. This dietary approach helps to ensure that the benefits of their physical activities are not undermined by adverse dietary effects.

14-Days Meal Plan

Below is a two-week meal plan designed for seniors participating in a chair yoga program, focusing on pre and post workout meals that will support their activity level and overall health. Each meal is selected to offer balanced nutrition, helping to enhance energy before workouts and aid recovery and muscle maintenance after workouts.

Week 1 Meal Plan

Day 1

- Pre Workout Meal: Greek Yogurt Parfait with Nuts and Honey
- Post Workout Meal: Chicken Salad with Avocado

Day 2

- Pre Workout Meal: Morning Oatmeal with Berries
- Post Workout Meal: Broccoli and Cheese Soup

Day 3

- Pre Workout Meal: Spinach and Feta Omelette
- Post Workout Meal: Baked Salmon with Dill

Day 4

- Pre Workout Meal: Apple Cinnamon Rice Pudding
- Post Workout Meal: Quinoa and Black Bean Salad

Day 5

- Pre Workout Meal: Tuna Salad on Whole Grain Bread
- Post Workout Meal: Beef and Vegetable Stir-Fry

Day 6
- Pre Workout Meal: Morning Oatmeal with Berries
- Post Workout Meal: Sweet Potato and Black Bean Chili

Day 7
- Pre Workout Meal: Greek Yogurt Parfait with Nuts and Honey
- Post Workout Meal: Lentil Soup

Week 2 Meal Plan

Day 8
- Pre Workout Meal: Spinach and Feta Omelette
- Post Workout Meal: Grilled Turkey and Vegetable Kebabs

Day 9
- Pre Workout Meal: Apple Cinnamon Rice Pudding
- Post Workout Meal: Roasted Vegetable Medley

Day 10
- Pre Workout Meal: Tuna Salad on Whole Grain Bread
- Post Workout Meal: Vegetable and Bean Soup

Day 11
- Pre Workout Meal: Morning Oatmeal with Berries
- Post Workout Meal: Chicken Salad with Avocado

Day 12
- Pre Workout Meal: Greek Yogurt Parfait with Nuts and Honey

- Post Workout Meal: Broccoli and Cheese Soup

Day 13
- Pre Workout Meal: Morning Oatmeal with Berries
- Post Workout Meal: Baked Salmon with Dill

Day 14
- Pre Workout Meal: Spinach and Feta Omelette
- Post Workout Meal: Sweet Potato and Black Bean Chili

This meal plan ensures that seniors receive a mix of carbohydrates for energy, protein for muscle maintenance, and fats for long-lasting energy and joint health, all crucial for those engaging in chair yoga. The timing of the meals helps maximize energy levels during workouts and recovery afterward.

PROGRESS TRACKER JOURNAL

The use of a progress tracker journal in your practice adds a deeply personal and reflective dimension to the process. This isn't just about maintaining physical health; it's about reclaiming independence and enjoying a fuller, more active life.

How would it feel to see those small daily victories over stiffness and immobility documented in your own handwriting? Picture the satisfaction of flipping back through the pages of your journal after a few weeks, witnessing the tangible progress you've made. Wouldn't it bring a sense of pride and accomplishment?

Benefits of Using the Progress Tracker Journal

- **- Accountability**: Regularly updating the journal encourages consistency and accountability, key components in building a sustainable exercise habit.
- **- Customization:** By tracking what works best for their bodies, seniors can customize exercises to maximize benefits and minimize risks.
- **- Recognition of Progress:** Visual evidence of progress in the journal boosts morale and motivation, especially on days when seniors might feel less inclined to exercise.
- **- Enhanced Communication with your doctor**: The detailed logs can be shared with healthcare providers, who can then offer more personalized advice based on the tracked data.

This progress tracker journal, used in conjunction with the chair yoga exercises, is an invaluable tool for you striving to improve your mobility, balance, and posture. By methodically documenting their journey, you not only see the physical benefits more clearly but also gain a sense of accomplishment and independence that enriches their quality of life.

CHAIR YOGA
PROGRESS TRACKER JOURNAL

WEEK ☐

WEEKLY GOALS

AFFIRMATION AND MOTIVATION

TO DO

- ☐
- ☐
- ☐
- ☐
- ☐
- ☐

SET BACKS:

	YES	NO
QUALITY SLEEP	☐	☐
PROPER HYDRATION	☐	☐

ACHIEVEMENTS

- ☐
- ☐
- ☐
- ☐
- ☐
- ☐

WEEKLY DISCOVERY:

IIMPROVED PLAN FOR A BETTER GOAL ACHIEVEMENTS IN THEFOLLOWING WEEK:

CHAIR YOGA
PROGRESS TRACKER JOURNAL

WEEK ☐

WEEKLY GOALS

AFFIRMATION AND MOTIVATION

TO DO

☐
☐
☐
☐
☐
☐

SET BACKS:

	YES	NO
QUALITY SLEEP	☐	☐
PROPER HYDRATION	☐	☐

ACHIEVEMENTS

☐
☐
☐
☐
☐
☐

WEEKLY DISCOVERY:

IIMPROVED PLAN FOR A BETTER GOAL ACHIEVEMENTS IN THEFOLLOWING WEEK:

CHAIR YOGA
PROGRESS TRACKER JOURNAL

WEEK ☐

WEEKLY GOALS

____

AFFIRMATION AND MOTIVATION

____

TO DO

☐ _______________
☐ _______________
☐ _______________
☐ _______________
☐ _______________
☐ _______________

SET BACKS:

	YES	NO
QUALITY SLEEP	☐	☐
PROPER HYDRATION	☐	☐

ACHIEVEMENTS

☐ _______________
☐ _______________
☐ _______________
☐ _______________
☐ _______________
☐ _______________

WEEKLY DISCOVERY:

IIMPROVED PLAN FOR A BETTER GOAL ACHIEVEMENTS IN THEFOLLOWING WEEK:

____

____

____

____

CHAIR YOGA
PROGRESS TRACKER JOURNAL

WEEK ☐

WEEKLY GOALS

AFFIRMATION AND MOTIVATION

TO DO

☐
☐
☐
☐
☐
☐

SET BACKS:

	YES	NO
QUALITY SLEEP	☐	☐
PROPER HYDRATION	☐	☐

ACHIEVEMENTS

☐
☐
☐
☐
☐
☐

WEEKLY DISCOVERY:

IIMPROVED PLAN FOR A BETTER GOAL ACHIEVEMENTS IN THEFOLLOWING WEEK:

CHAIR YOGA
PROGRESS TRACKER JOURNAL

WEEK ☐

WEEKLY GOALS

____

AFFIRMATION AND MOTIVATION

____

TO DO

☐
☐
☐
☐
☐
☐

SET BACKS:

	YES	NO
QUALITY SLEEP	☐	☐
PROPER HYDRATION	☐	☐

ACHIEVEMENTS

☐
☐
☐
☐
☐
☐

WEEKLY DISCOVERY:

IIMPROVED PLAN FOR A BETTER GOAL ACHIEVEMENTS IN THEFOLLOWING WEEK:

____

CHAIR YOGA
PROGRESS TRACKER JOURNAL

WEEK ☐

WEEKLY GOALS

AFFIRMATION AND MOTIVATION

TO DO

☐
☐
☐
☐
☐
☐

SET BACKS:

	YES	NO
QUALITY SLEEP	☐	☐
PROPER HYDRATION	☐	☐

ACHIEVEMENTS

☐
☐
☐
☐
☐
☐

WEEKLY DISCOVERY:

IIMPROVED PLAN FOR A BETTER GOAL ACHIEVEMENTS IN THEFOLLOWING WEEK:

CHAIR YOGA
PROGRESS TRACKER JOURNAL

WEEK ☐

WEEKLY GOALS

AFFIRMATION AND MOTIVATION

TO DO

☐
☐
☐
☐
☐
☐

ACHIEVEMENTS

☐
☐
☐
☐
☐
☐

SET BACKS:

	YES	NO
QUALITY SLEEP	☐	☐
PROPER HYDRATION	☐	☐

WEEKLY DISCOVERY:

IIMPROVED PLAN FOR A BETTER GOAL ACHIEVEMENTS IN THEFOLLOWING WEEK:

CHAIR YOGA
PROGRESS TRACKER JOURNAL   WEEK ☐

WEEKLY GOALS

AFFIRMATION AND MOTIVATION

TO DO

☐
☐
☐
☐
☐
☐

ACHIEVEMENTS

☐
☐
☐
☐
☐
☐

SET BACKS:

YES	NO
QUALITY SLEEP ☐	☐
PROPER HYDRATION ☐	☐

WEEKLY DISCOVERY:

IIMPROVED PLAN FOR A BETTER GOAL ACHIEVEMENTS IN THEFOLLOWING WEEK:

CHAIR YOGA
PROGRESS TRACKER JOURNAL

WEEK ☐

WEEKLY GOALS

____

AFFIRMATION AND MOTIVATION

____

TO DO

- ☐ __________
- ☐ __________
- ☐ __________
- ☐ __________
- ☐ __________
- ☐ __________

SET BACKS:

☐ (box)

	YES	NO
QUALITY SLEEP	☐	☐
PROPER HYDRATION	☐	☐

ACHIEVEMENTS

- ☐ __________
- ☐ __________
- ☐ __________
- ☐ __________
- ☐ __________
- ☐ __________

WEEKLY DISCOVERY:

☐ (box)

IIMPROVED PLAN FOR A BETTER GOAL ACHIEVEMENTS IN THEFOLLOWING WEEK:

____

CHAIR YOGA
PROGRESS TRACKER JOURNAL

WEEK ☐

WEEKLY GOALS

AFFIRMATION AND MOTIVATION

TO DO

- ☐
- ☐
- ☐
- ☐
- ☐
- ☐

ACHIEVEMENTS

- ☐
- ☐
- ☐
- ☐
- ☐
- ☐

SET BACKS:

	YES	NO
QUALITY SLEEP	☐	☐
PROPER HYDRATION	☐	☐

WEEKLY DISCOVERY:

IIMPROVED PLAN FOR A BETTER GOAL ACHIEVEMENTS IN THEFOLLOWING WEEK:

CHAIR YOGA
PROGRESS TRACKER JOURNAL

WEEK ☐

WEEKLY GOALS

AFFIRMATION AND MOTIVATION

TO DO

- ☐
- ☐
- ☐
- ☐
- ☐
- ☐

SET BACKS:

	YES	NO
QUALITY SLEEP	☐	☐
PROPER HYDRATION	☐	☐

ACHIEVEMENTS

- ☐
- ☐
- ☐
- ☐
- ☐
- ☐

WEEKLY DISCOVERY:

IIMPROVED PLAN FOR A BETTER GOAL ACHIEVEMENTS IN THEFOLLOWING WEEK:

CHAIR YOGA
PROGRESS TRACKER JOURNAL

WEEK ☐

WEEKLY GOALS

AFFIRMATION AND MOTIVATION

TO DO

☐
☐
☐
☐
☐
☐

SET BACKS:

	YES	NO
QUALITY SLEEP	☐	☐
PROPER HYDRATION	☐	☐

ACHIEVEMENTS

☐
☐
☐
☐
☐
☐

WEEKLY DISCOVERY:

IIMPROVED PLAN FOR A BETTER GOAL ACHIEVEMENTS IN THEFOLLOWING WEEK:

CONCLUSION

As we come to the close of this book, I hope you have found it not only beneficial but also enriching and enjoyable. Thank you for choosing this guide to accompany you on a truly remarkable journey towards improved mobility, balance, posture and help you lose unnecessary weight . Each page you turned and each exercise you performed has been a step towards reclaiming your independence and enhancing your quality of life.

Did you enjoy your experience with this program? I would love to hear how this journey has impacted you, both physically and emotionally. Your feedback is invaluable and can inspire others to journey on their own paths to better health and wellness.

Final Advice:

Keep moving forward. The end of this book doesn't mean the end of the road. I encourage you to revisit the exercises that you found most beneficial and to continue incorporating them into your daily routine. Remember, consistency is key to maintaining the gains you've achieved. Here's to many more days of improved health, flexibility, and peace of mind. You've proven that it's never too late to start feeling better and living more fully.

Thank you once again for allowing this book to be a part of your health and wellness journey. Keep striving, keep stretching, and keep shining in your golden years!

Thank you for choosing **"10-Minute Chair Yoga for Seniors Over 60"** as your guide to a healthier, more vibrant life. We hope you have found the exercises and information in this book both inspiring and beneficial as you continue on your journey towards greater mobility, balance, and independence.

Your feedback is incredibly valuable to us and to others considering embarking on their own path to wellness. If you've enjoyed the book or have insights to share about your experience with the 28-day challenge, please take a moment to leave a positive feedback on Amazon. Your feedback not only helps us to improve but also inspires others to take the first step towards a healthier lifestyle.

Leaving a review is easy:
1. Go to the page where you purchased the book.
2. Scroll down to the 'Customer Feedback' section.
3. Click on 'Write a Customer Feedback.
4. Rate the book and write your thoughts.

Thank you once again for your trust and commitment to your health. Remember, every small step counts towards a larger journey of well-being. Keep moving, keep stretching, and keep thriving!

With gratitude,